# A Little More Than Perfect

# A Little More Than

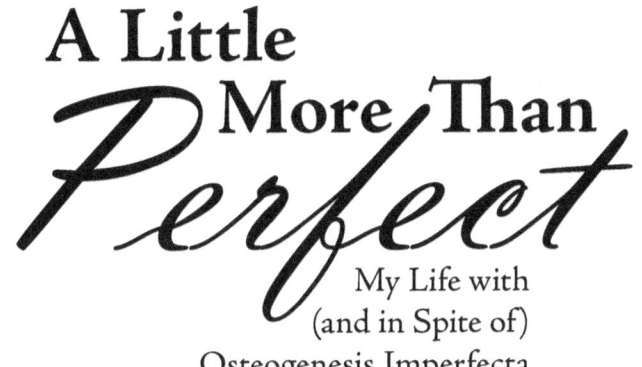

Perfect

My Life with
(and in Spite of)
Osteogenesis Imperfecta

*Heather Anderson*

iUniverse, Inc.
New York   Bloomington

**A Little More Than Perfect**
**My Life with (and in Spite of) Osteogenesis Imperfecta**

iUniverse books may be ordered through booksellers or by contacting:

iUniverse
1663 Liberty Drive
Bloomington, IN 47403
www.iuniverse.com
1-800-Authors (1-800-288-4677)

ISBN: 978-0-595-51087-0 (sc)
ISBN: 978-0-595-50348-3 (dj)
ISBN: 978-0-595-61760-9 (ebk)

Printed in the United States of America

iUniverse rev. date: 02/08/2010

I dedicate this book to my parents, Margaret and Eric Anderson,
for showing me that life is beautiful
and
for teaching me to live to the beat of my own rhythm.

# Contents

# *Acknowledgment*

I once met a very spiritual woman who told me, "You are an amazing person, and I feel honored to have met you. I am in awe of you, but you could never have become the woman you are today without an amazing person behind you."

That amazing person who has supported me all my life is my mom. I wrote this book to honor my mom, who gave me the greatest gift one could ever receive. She continues to show me in all that she does that I was born absolutely perfect, as is everyone else with whom I share this world. We are born the way that God wants us to be, and when we grow up with that knowledge, we have the power within ourselves to move mountains.

I sometimes wonder if my mother realizes the importance of her life. I know that when I was born with osteogenesis imperfecta (OI), the enormity of the responsibility shook her world to the core, but through the experience of caring for a child with OI, I believe that she found the true meaning of her life. Suddenly, none of the mundane things in life were important. She knew that all that mattered was living *in* the moment and *for* the moment.

She has touched the lives of many people, and I believe that she has lived a life full of meaning and accomplishment. I hope that I can become even half the woman that my mother is. I am so grateful to be able to call her Mom.

# *Introduction*

I'm forty-five years old, and I've had more than a hundred fractures in my life … so far. Am I clumsy? Do I have a dangerous job? Have I been in some kind of serious accident? No. I have osteogenesis imperfecta (OI), a genetic disorder that makes my bones as brittle as glass. When I was about seven or eight years old, Mom and I went to see the Ice Capades at the Fort William Gardens in our hometown of Thunder Bay, Ontario. It was December, so we were bundled up in our big winter coats. As Mom and I settled into our seats, she gently tugged on the sleeve of my coat to shake my arm out. Just that slight tug on my coat sleeve resulted in a broken arm. There we were, in the middle of a packed arena, me screaming and crying in pain and the people around us wondering what had happened. Mom wrapped my coat around my arm as best she could to support it, and then, carrying me in her arms, she struggled to make her way through the crowd, phone my Dad, and wait to make yet another trip to the hospital.

Episodes like this were a regular occurrence in our family. I think that's one of the reasons I wanted to tell my story. The other reason is that for as long as I can remember, I've wanted to understand why we are here and why things happen to us in life. For many years, I thought about writing a book, but as the years passed, I wasn't quite sure what I wanted to write about. However, as my life evolved, I began to imagine my book as a personal interpretation of the lessons that life has taught me.

The fact that a fracture can be caused by something as simple as a sneeze is unimaginable to most people, but that's how easily my bones can break. Many times, people have asked me whether I'm angry about having been born with OI. My answer has always been "No." Of course, I endured some tough times emotionally as I was growing up, but I can honestly say that I have always felt blessed. My life's journey has presented me with some wonderful experiences and opportunities, and I feel enriched by the people who have crossed my path, the challenges that I have faced, and the intense soul searching that has come from living with a disability. Life has taught me that a disability is merely a state of mind.

Over the years, people have asked me, "Why are you so small?" or they've made condescending comments like, "Your life must be difficult. I feel so sorry for you." Yes, I am small; yes, life is difficult at times, as it is for everyone; and no, people don't ever have to feel sorry for me. Instead, my life is a testimony to the human spirit's ability to endure the worst challenges imaginable.

My favorite quote is, "Born a little more than perfect into a world a little less than perfect" (author unknown). I hope that readers of this book will feel a little better about life, accept the lessons of life, and appreciate all their experiences on this earth.

"May you have enough happiness to make you sweet, enough trials to make you strong, enough sorrow to keep you humble, and enough hope to make you happy" (author unknown).

# Part One

## My Story

# Chapter 1

## *The Beginning*

My name is Heather Anderson, and I was born on September 26, 1963, in Thunder Bay, Ontario, Canada, to Margaret and Eric Anderson at St. Joseph's General Hospital. My parents were married in 1954 in a quiet ceremony in St. John's Anglican Church, with Reverand. S. Maitland Craymer officiating. A reception followed at my mother's parents' home. My mother was a strikingly lovely, pencil-thin twenty-seven-year-old auburn-haired beauty. My father was a dashing thirty-one-year-old man with a medium build. He had warm hazel eyes and

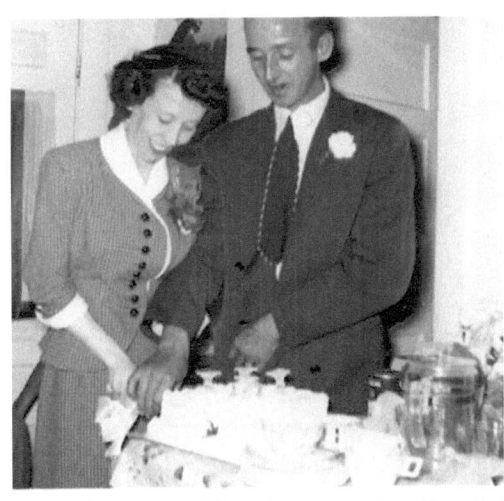

*Mom & Dad's wedding day, September 30, 1954*

dark brown wavy hair. Both of my parents had impeccable taste in fashion and were very stylish. Dad never left the house without shiny shoes. The marriage announcement read like this: "The bride chose a navy blue pinstriped wool dressmaker suit with a fitted jacket with white corded silk collar and cored silk cuffs on the three-quarter length sleeves. Her small pillbox hat of navy velvet had a nose veil and she wore white kid gloves and navy suede pumps. American Beauty roses were in her corsage."

After a short honeymoon, my parents purchased their first home and immediately began their family. Sheila was born March 10, 1955; Carol was next on July 6, 1958, and then Clifford on April 4, 1961. I

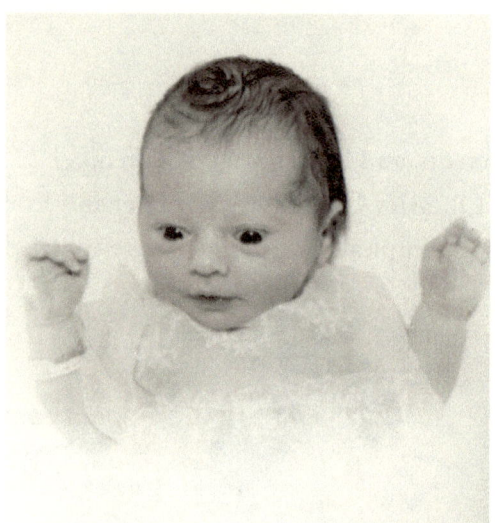

*Heather's first photo, September 26, 1963*

was the last one, born on September 26, 1963. In those days, fathers were not permitted in the delivery room, and mothers were sedated during delivery, not fully aware of whether they had delivered a boy or girl until they were brought back to their rooms and the sedation had begun to wear off. Babies did not sleep with their mothers. All of the babies were kept in the nursery and were brought to their mothers only for feeding. They were then immediately taken back to the nursery, where the nurses cared for them until the next feeding. Visiting hours were very strict, and no one was allowed in before or after the posted visiting hours. St. Joseph's Hospital was very strict, as it was completely managed by nuns. Mothers stayed in the hospital for at least a week before being released. Shortly after I was born, the nurse entered my mother's room and said, "Mrs. Anderson, you have a healthy baby girl." The nurse smiled and told my mother, "She has brown hair and brown eyes and weighs just over five pounds." Mom remembers feeling relieved and overjoyed that she and my dad had a new daughter to bring home to their three other children. They, of course, were unaware that the joy and happiness they were feeling was not to last long and that their faith would be tested to the limit. Their world was about to turn upside down. Two days after my birth, Dr. Hawkins and Sister Leila Greco from St. Joseph's came into my mother's hospital room. Dr Hawkins was the first to speak. "Mrs. Anderson," he began, his tone matching the serious expression on his face. "There's something we need to discuss with you about the baby, Heather."

Her voice trembling, my mother asked them, "What do you mean? Is there something wrong with my baby?"

Dr. Hawkins told her, "We think that she may have a very rare bone condition called osteogenesis imperfecta."

"Osteo what? Wait a minute! You said that my baby was fine. You told me that just yesterday. What are you saying? This can't be!" My mother screamed, and tears began to roll down her face.

Sister Greco stepped toward my mom, reaching out to take her hand. She said, "Mrs. Anderson, I realize that this is devastating and heartbreaking news for any parent to hear, but let's wait until Dr. Mutrie, the orthopedic doctor, examines her, and then we will know for sure where things stand." Dr. Hawkins lowered his head, and except for the sounds of my mother's sobbing, a heavy silence fell over the room.

Mom tried to pull herself together as best as

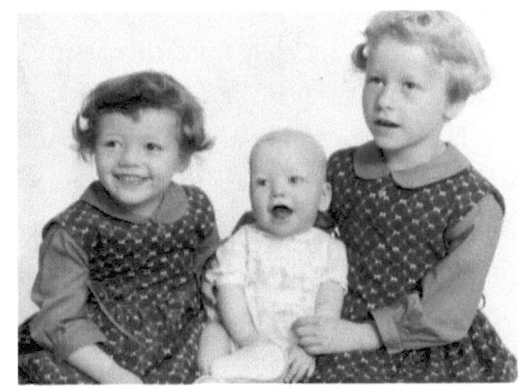

*L. to R. Carol, Clifford, and Sheila, 1963*

she could, and then she dialed my dad at work to let him know that he was needed at the hospital immediately. When Dad arrived my mother told him what was going on. They were in a state of complete shock. They sat holding each other, not saying a word. A million thoughts raced through both their minds, but each did not want to upset the other, and both hoped that they would soon have all of the facts.

Just then, the door to my mother's hospital room suddenly opened, and Dr. Hawkins, Dr. Mutrie, and Sister Greco entered. A deafening, eerie stillness filled the room. Dr. Mutrie was the first to speak, in a tone of voice that was serious yet somehow comforting. He said, "Mr. and Mrs. Anderson, your baby has been diagnosed with osteogenesis imperfecta. OI is a genetic disorder characterized by bones that break easily, often from little or no apparent cause."

My parents listened with great intensity, hanging on to his every word. Dr, Mutrie continued, "There is a commonly used classification system of different types of OI that helps describe how severely a person with OI is affected. For example, a person may have just a few or as many as several hundred fractures in a lifetime.

Mom said, "How severely has our baby been affected?"

Dr. Mutrie replied, "At this point we are not sure; she was not born with any fractures. That's a good sign. We will have to wait and see over time."

His voice cracking, my father asked, "How many people are affected with OI and what is the cause?"

Dr. Mutrie replied, "The number of people affected with OI is unknown. The best estimate suggests a minimum of 20,000 and possibly as many as 50,000. OI is caused by genetic defects that affect the body's ability to make strong bones. In dominant (classical) OI, a person has too little type I collagen or a poor quality of type I collagen due to a mutation in one of the type I collagen genes. Collagen is the major protein of the body's connective tissue. This is part of the framework that bones are formed around. In recessive OI, mutations in other genes interfere with collagen production. The result in all cases is fragile bones that break easily."

In that single moment their lives had changed forever. My father asked in a quiet voice, "Is there a cure?"

Dr. Mutrie continued. "There is not yet a cure for OI. Treatment is directed toward preventing or controlling the symptoms, maximizing independent mobility, and developing optimal bone mass and muscle strength. You will need to care for the fractures as they happen; extensive surgical and dental procedures may be needed, and physical therapy is often recommended."

My mother asked, "Will she ever be able to walk?"

Dr. Mutrie replied, "She may need to use a wheelchair, braces, or other mobility aids, although not all people with OI need aids. It will depend on the severity of the OI. At this point we will have to wait and see."

My father spoke. "What do we do from this point on?"

Dr. Hawkins replied, "You are to care for her as if she were your best china."

For my mother, that was the day her whole world began to fall apart. She can still recall what happened that day. She heard them explain what it was, but she couldn't understand how such an unimaginable condition could happen to her little girl. What were they talking about? What was going to happen to her baby girl? In dazed confusion, she and Dad brought me home a week after my birth. Neither of them had the slightest idea of the challenges that the years would bring.

Dad went back to work after Mom and I were released from the hospital, when I was about a week old. Fathers were not able to take time off in 1963 to stay home and help with the new baby unless without pay, something that was not feasible for my parents.

The first fracture happened a week after I was home from the hospital. Mom took me to the doctor for my first checkup. The simple, normal infant behaviors of crying and waving my arms resulted in a broken collarbone, the first of so many fractures to come. Back in those days the public health nurse would stop by to check in on new mothers.

She began coming to our home on a regular basis, trying to offer some comfort and support to my mother. Mom remembers saying to her, "I feel completely helpless because no one can tell me or show me how to care for my baby. I am completely on my own. The days are passing, and I am falling into a world of lonely sorrow."

My sisters were both attending school at this point, but my brother was only three years old. My maternal grandmother and grandfather helped to care for him while Mom and I were still in the hospital, but once we were home he was home all day with Mom and me while Dad was at work. We were fortunate that our Nanny and Grandpa (on my Mom's side) lived just three blocks away from our home. My grandpa was of Irish ancestry, and Nanny was born in Quebec. As I got older, I remember my grandpa walking down to our house every day for a little visit until he could no longer walk the three blocks. Nanny also came by often.

Nanny was about sixty when I was born. She was a fairly large woman with a happy and outgoing personality. She had bright red hair when she was young, and I remember her always telling us that when she met Grandpa he used to call her Carrot Top. My grandpa was ten years older than Nanny, so he would have been seventy years old when I was born. He was a small, slender, and very gentle person, quite the opposite of my Nanny.

My mom took after her father, except for her mother's red hair. Mom's only sibling was a brother, Kenny, who was five years younger. My Uncle Kenny and Auntie Pat were quite close to our family. They eventually ended up having eight children, which meant they were very busy. My dad's parents came to Canada from Sweden before they were married. Dad's father passed away at a young age, when Dad was only four years old. His mother, a nurse, remarried after Dad's father passed away, but my Dad and his stepfather were never very close.

Unfortunately Dad's mother passed away when she also was quite young, when my dad was in his late twenties. Dad had three sisters:

Dolly, Betty, and Greta. They moved away from home when we were quite young. Aunt Betty moved out west, and Aunt Greta moved up north to work in a bush camp. We never saw too much of them after they moved. Although my siblings and I never had the opportunity to know our paternal grandparents, our maternal grandparents made sure that they spoiled us.

My maternal grandmother loved me and would drop by to help my mother, but she couldn't cope with everything that was happening. She was a very excitable person. When she heard my cries of pain from yet another broken bone, she became afraid that she would hurt me if she picked me up. And she couldn't give my mother the emotional support that she so desperately needed. Grandma would say to my mother, "I can't stand to hear her screaming. I don't know how you deal with all the crying." Mom's answer to that was, "I don't have a choice. I don't like to hear my baby screaming from another fracture any more than you do, but someone has to be strong to help her." As much as Mom loved her mother, she felt that she was just no help to her.

Each day was worse than the one before. My bones continued to fracture, and constant visits to the doctor became a normal part of our lives. Doctors couldn't do much for me other than support the injured limbs as much as possible to help them heal properly.

Aside from the public health nurse stopping by, Mom pretty much handled us kids on her own. Being the mother of three other children meant that she was experienced with the demands of a new baby, but getting used to caring for a baby as fragile as glass was something else. Mom said, "The doctor always told me to make sure I kept your fractured limb straight when wrapping it so that the bone would grow straight, so I would wrap and unwrap the limb over and over again. I was so afraid of doing it wrong—not too loose, not too tight. My God, I must have driven myself crazy over that!"

Dad worked as the truck driver for all the local grain elevators with the Saskatchewan Wheat Pool. His shift was 5:00 AM to 1:00 PM

Monday to Friday. After he got home he would have lunch and then go out to his workshop. He was a self-taught carpenter and remodeled many people's kitchens in our hometown to make extra money for the family. So for the most part Mom was our primary caregiver; Dad had his hands full making money to support the family. My oldest sister Sheila was eight years old when I was born. She was a great help to Mom, and I believe that Mom really came to rely on her over the years. Carol, who was five years old when I was born, helped out as much as she could.

Mom can remember the moment when everything changed for her and a weight lifted from her shoulders. It happened just before my first Christmas. The tree wasn't up yet, the house wasn't decorated as usual, and there were no gifts. Between September and December, Mom had been in a daze, going through the motions of daily living, but she had felt numb since my birth. Instead of the sounds of joy, the house was filled with the screams of a baby in constant pain. Many days, Dad came home to find me screaming from a new fracture and Mom crying from fatigue and helplessness.

Just before Christmas, my brother told my grandmother, "We're not having Christmas this year, Nanny, because Mom is really sad about the baby." My grandmother told my Mom, "Margaret, I know that you are struggling to make sense of the situation since Heather was born, and I know that I have not been able to give you the support that you need, but in some way you have to pull yourself out of this depression, for the other children. Clifford told me today that there won't be Christmas at his home this year because Mommy is so sad about the baby." Mom lowered her head and sobbed. "What am I doing? I'm of no help to Heather or my other children by acting this way. From this day on, I am not going to let OI rule our lives. We will get through this challenge the best way we can. I will make sure that my children enjoy everything that life has to offer and never again will I allow this to change our lives. Everything happens for a reason, and

I am going to turn this situation into a reason to fight. I will find the strength to overcome any obstacle in our way."

From that day forward, something inside my mother changed, and she began to realize that her depression was of no help to my siblings or me. She became determined that we would be a normal family and get through this challenge the best way we could. We would deal with each obstacle as it came along. Even though there were tough times and many more fractures ahead, we never again looked at or thought of OI in the same way. As the years passed, that day would serve as a reminder that believing that we can change things can and will make wonderful things happen.

# Chapter 2

## *A New Reality*

There had been a period of adjusting and accepting for everyone involved as we entered month five of our new reality. As they continually explained my condition to family and friends, my parents were beginning to feel like broken records, stuck in one spot. My mother recalls telling her neighbor Annabel, "At times I feel as though I have lived a lifetime in the past four months since Heather was born. Caring for her has been more difficult than I could have ever imagined. I cannot begin to tell you how deeply my heart is aching. I have to constantly remind myself of the promise I made to my children that we will get through this." Annabel reached out to touch my mother's hand and replied, "You will get through this, Margaret! You just need to have faith that everything will be fine." The blank stare on my mother's face had replaced her once happy and youthful smile. She lowered her head and sighed as if to say, "I have nothing left to give."

When my mom would bath me, she told me, "I would heat olive oil and gently rub your legs and feet because both of your feet turned inward and your legs were crunched tight up to your chest. I had to wrap your diaper over your knees because I could not get it between your knees and chest. I was determined that I would massage your little legs gently until they straightened out." Eventually, after months and months of my Mom's olive oil massages, my legs began to release from their tight position, and my feet no longer turned inward. Mom said, "I think you really enjoyed it when I rubbed the warm oil. You would just stare off into space."

Once my legs began to release from the fetal position and my feet turned around the right way, it was hard to imagine that I had such a horrific condition. I was average size and weight, had ten perfect little fingers and ten perfect little toes. The only tell-tale sign was what the doctor noticed at birth that made him aware that something might be wrong: I had blue sclera, which is the white part of our eyes. People born with OI have blue sclera. I recall over the years Mom saying, "When you were born the whites of your eyes were blue like the sky on a perfect summer day and with your dark brown eye color, they were so beautiful." Leave it to Mom to find the beauty in my brown eyes being blue. Over the years the blue sclera began to fade to a whiter shade.

By the end of the first year, the reality of just how fragile my bones were had came full circle for my parents. The fractures were constant, sometimes two in one day. One day Mom had put me in my crib while she got my sisters and brother ready for school. I was fussing and crying, so Sheila gave me her pencil case to play with. I began shaking it to hear the pencils rattling inside, but then I dropped it on my stomach. The result was a broken pelvis.

Often, the day my mother removed a sling from my healed arm, my leg would be broken by the evening. The only bonus with OI is that bones heal as easily as they fracture, usually within two weeks. Back when I was young, doctors still made house calls. As time went on and my parents became more comfortable with dealing with each fracture, they would call our family doctor to come to our house and set the leg or arm, whichever it may be. Sometimes with a leg fracture, it was necessary to put the leg in traction. Rather than putting me in the hospital each time, Dad told the doctor, "I will make the traction on her crib. Just tell me how I need to make it and how heavy the weights need to be." The doctor showed my dad how it should be and off to his workshop he went to make a homemade traction. Tractions have a bit of a weight on the end of a pulley system that holds the leg straight and keeps tension on it in order to allow the leg to heal proper. Dad spared me from having to spend time in the hospital over and over again. Mom always recalled one stormy winter's night when Dad was working and she was home alone with us kids. She said, "I called Dr. Schiewe to tell him that you had fractured your leg. He said, 'I'll be right there, Margaret.' Big snowflakes were falling when he arrived. By the time he was finished setting your leg and getting you comfortable, the wind had gotten up and visibility was very poor. Shortly after he left I heard a knock at the door. I went to the door, and there was the doctor. He said, 'Margaret, I seem to be stuck on some ice. Do you have sand that I can spread under my tire?'" Mom said, "I'll go to the garage and see if Eric has some out there." Mom bundled herself up and told the other children, "I'm going to the garage to get some sand for the doctor. He's stuck on a patch of ice. Please keep an eye on your sister and don't wake her up. She just settled down. and I want her to get some rest." The other kids said, "Okay, Mom." Mom said, "Between the doctor pushing the car and the sand I threw under his tire, he finally got off the ice and was on his way."

Mom was bothered by how the nurses would look at her each time she brought me to the doctor's office or emergency room with a new fracture. Mom said, "When we came across a nurse that was not aware of your condition, she would give me a look that could have killed, thinking that I caused your fracture." With today's greater awareness and intolerance of child abuse, everyone with a child with OI is advised to carry a letter from their doctor explaining that the child has OI. Since there are so many variations of OI, often the child may look perfectly average on the outside, but the bones inside are still very fragile.

I remember Mom saying, "You were such a good baby, we could spend all day between the doctor's office and getting X-rays and you would scream in pain, but once we got home and I got you comfortable,

I would feed you and you would eat every drop. You never fussed at meal time, no matter how hard a day you had."

I often think about what my parents, particularly my mother, went through during those years. As just one example, Mom dreaded changing my diapers because she knew that she would have to move one of my fractured limbs. Each time that she changed me, my cries of pain would resonate through the house. Twenty-four hours a day she endured every painful moment along with me. When we talk about that time now, it seems surreal to us—almost as if it never really happened, as if it were a novel or a story that someone made up. But this *is* my life story.

Life went on. Mom and Dad maintained as normal an existence for all of us kids as they possibly could. I'm not sure how my siblings handled the situation, but they seemed to adjust. Kids are far more adaptable than most adults, quickly learning that they had to be careful when holding me or playing with me. Since there are eight years between my sister Sheila and I, she was able to quickly learn how to handle me in order to help Mom out. They all sacrificed a great deal during their young lives.

Because I never spent any time in the hospital and Mom was home and able to be there for the other kids as well, our family life was fairly normal, except for the fractures. I imagine Mom's day was quite full and very busy, but she was there with all of us, and she managed to hold down the fort even during the storms. Despite the difficulties, I remember our home as being quite happy and lively. My siblings were busy coming and going between school and friends. Everyone found a way to accept the new reality and continue on with life.

There was a grocery store about a block down the road from where we lived. Many times Sheila would go grocery shopping for Mom when it was just too hectic at home for Mom to get out and Dad was busy working. One time Sheila came running in the house from the grocery store crying and all upset, and she said, "Mom, I lost the grocery money that you gave me. I was looking at the meat counter and I dropped it. I'm so sorry!" as she gasped for breath through her tears. She thought that Mom was going to be really mad because she lost all the grocery money. Mom said, "What's wrong? Everything will be fine. We will phone the store and see if anyone has found the money." So Mom called and spoke to the manager, and he said to send Sheila back and he would help her look. Off Sheila went, red-faced and still clearly upset. A while later she came busting through the door yelling, "Mom, Mom, I found the money! The store manager found it in between the meat at the meat counter. I guess I put it down while I was looking and then forgot to pick it up." From that day on Sheila made sure she never put her money down again. There were times that my siblings were forced to grow up a little faster because of me. Mom needed their help sometimes when Dad could not be there, so the other kids needed to take on responsibilities at young ages.

My parents never went out much, only when they had to. Nanny and Grandpa would come and stay with us once in awhile if my parents had to go somewhere important together, like parent-teacher interviews at the school. Other than that we never had a babysitter; either Mom or Dad was home with us. Mom was afraid to leave me with anyone, and I'm sure most people were afraid to be left alone with me.

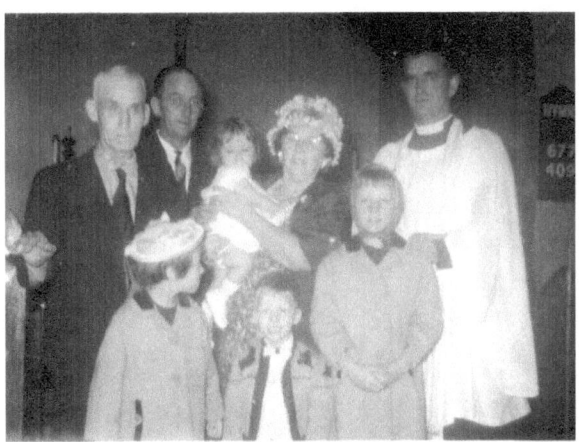

*Back row: Grandpa Grattan, Dad,*
*Nanny Grattan (holding Heather), Rev. Lumley.*
*Front row: Carol, Clifford and Sheila, 1965*

My parents were quite good friends with the neighbors across the street from our home, Annabel and Leo

Paavola. Their three children Lisa, Wendy, and Larry were the same ages as my siblings, so they played back and forth together a lot. Mom often recalls the time Mrs. Paavola invited Mom over for tea, and they

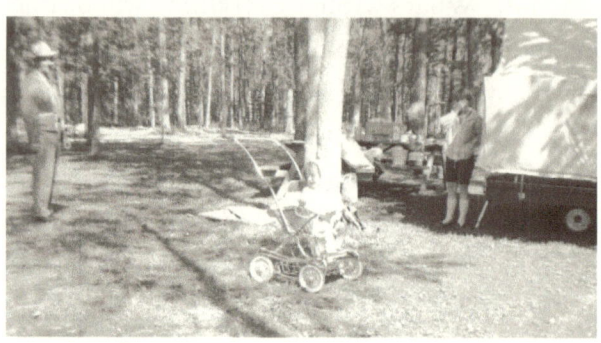

*L. to R. Dad, Heather in carriage, Sheila, camping trip 1966*

were talking about how things were going. Mrs. Paavola said, "Margaret, do you realize this is the first time you have been out of your house for enjoyment in six months?" Mom

laughed and said, "Has it really been that long since I came over for tea with you?" Annabel replied, "I don't know how you do it, Margaret." Just knowing that someone understood helped my mom find the strength to keep going, one day at a time.

They always talked and laughed about the time Mrs. Paavola was pregnant with Larry. Her husband was out of town at the time, and she called to my Mom and said, "Margaret, I'm having the baby, is Eric home? I need him to take me to the hospital." At the time my dad was out in the backyard pouring cement for a sidewalk. So off he went, cement-covered clothes and all, to bring Mrs. Paavo-

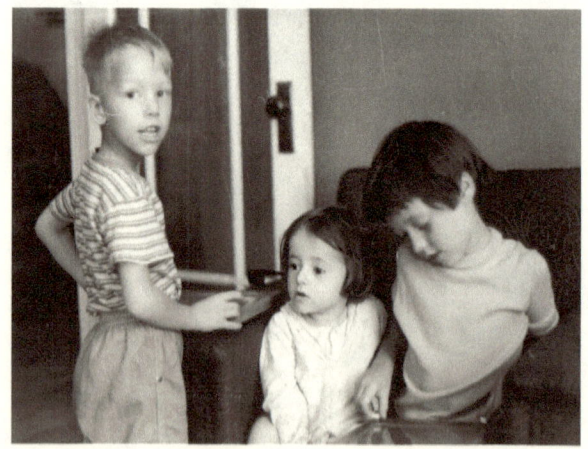

*L. to R. Clifford, Heather (age 3) and Carol*

la to the hospital. Despite all the hard times, there were equally as many good times.

In between the fractures, we went on outings as a family. We camped a lot; as long as I did not need to be in traction, my parents could still bundle me up, and off we would go. I began crawling and trying to walk by pulling myself up along furniture at the same age any average child would, but my parents had to watch that I never fell or bumped myself to hard. By age three I had started to learn to ride my tricycle. I was able to turn the peddles just as long as someone stayed close beside me so I would not fall off.

My dad was doing carpentry work for a young couple. One day, he noticed that their son was outside playing on his scooter. When Dad showed an interest, the boy's father asked why, so my Dad explained, "My little daughter is going to be four years old and was born with a rare bone condition and is unable to walk. That little scooter would be just the thing for her to get around." Right then and there, the father said to his son, "This man's little girl was born with very fragile bones and she is not able to walk like you. How do you feel about us giving your scooter to him so his daughter is able to get around like you can without the scooter?" The child agreed, and they gave it to my dad.

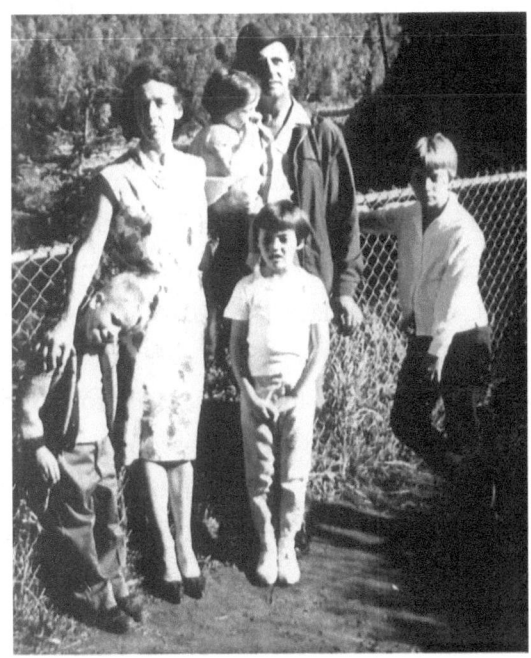

*Family photo taken at Kakabeka Falls. L. to R. Clifford, Mom, Dad (holding Heather), Carol in front, and Sheila, summer of 1967.*

When Dad came home, I remember he sat me in the scooter, and I started going around the house. I'm not sure where the family had got that scooter from; none of us had ever seen this type of scooter before. I would compare it to a baby walker. It was painted red. I'd sit in the seat and push the cart with my feet, I remember. From that day on I used that little scooter all the time. The generosity shown by that little boy and his father had a tremendous impact on our lives. What one child thought of as a toy was the gift of freedom and mobility to me. One small gesture of kindness can make all the difference in the world to someone.

Mom and I were unable to find a picture of it. Mom said, "When you were young I never took a lot of pictures because I had my hands full, and taking pictures was not exactly the first thing on my mind." When I asked my siblings if they remembered it, they all said, "Yes! Whatever happened to that little cart?"

I remember being so excited and happy about starting school. Mom was very worried about sending me to school, afraid that the other children might pick on me or that I could get hurt. The public health nurse calmed many of my mother's fears when she told her, "She's ready to start school." In her heart, Mom knew it too. So in the first week of September, just before my fifth birthday, I was registered to start school at Black Bay Road School. I didn't have a wheelchair when I started kindergarten; I'm not sure why. I think it just wasn't usual in the 1960s to provide wheelchairs for children. So off to school I went that year with my little red scooter. Mom laughs when she recalls that first day of school. She brought me into the classroom, and the teacher showed us around and took us to our table. I sat with a small group of other children around a little round table. Each table was named after a bird. I sat at the Blue Bird table.

Some of the other children cried and clung to their mothers. Apparently, I just turned around, waved, and said, "Bye, Mom." Right then my mother knew that I was ready for school. I enjoyed learning new things, and I especially loved doing arts and crafts. Even before I went to school, I used to spend hours coloring. Mom still has many of those pictures. She once told me that by age two, I was coloring inside the lines of the pictures.

The board of education arranged and paid for a taxi to pick up me up and bring me to school each day, as well as return me back home. Mom would come in the morning with us in the cab to make sure I got into class. At the end of the day Sheila would wait with me until the cab came, and she would put me in the cab. Sheila was in her last year of public school that year, grade 8. Sheila's friends and her boyfriend John would wait with us after school for the taxicab to arrive. I remember coming home some days crying, and Mom would ask me, "Why are you crying?" I would never say why, so she asked Sheila. "Why is Heather crying some days when she gets home?" Sheila would say, "I don't know why." Mom would ask if something happened, and Sheila would say, "No, I don't know why she keeps doing that." Finally I told my Mom that I was crying because when Sheila and I were waiting for the taxicab to arrive, sometimes her friends (who were much bigger than me) would wait with us and would push each other around, playing. I was scared that one of them was going to fall on me and I would get hurt. Once I finally confessed to what was wrong, Mom made sure that Sheila and her friends did not do any pushing and shoving when I was around. I had become consciously aware of how easily I could get hurt.

I made a lot of friends during the year: Carol, Cathy, Harry, Arnold, and Bradley, just to mention a few. We all played together a lot that year after school and on weekends, as well as over the course of the summer. Harry would come to my house all most every day that summer, I remember, and we played outside in the yard in my sandbox. That was one of my favorite pastimes.

I always had a big phobia about bugs. I remember playing in the sand one time by myself, and I saw some ants coming toward me. I started screaming and crying as I tried to get away from them. Mom came running outside and said, "What's wrong!" I said, "The ants are coming after me and I hurt my ankle trying to get way." Mom said, "Why are you so afraid of a little ant? You are much bigger than the ant." I ended up with a fractured ankle; my fear of bugs never improved much over the years.

I'll never forget Bradley. He was the cutest little white-haired boy in school and my best friend in kindergarten. He came to my house to play almost every day. Shortly after becoming friends with him, I broke my leg, but Bradley did not understand what that meant. His mother finally called Mom and told her that Bradley really needed to see me so that he could understand what it meant to break a leg. Later that day a knock came at the door. Mom answered. I heard her say, "Hello, Bradley, come on in and see Heather." Bradley approached with caution, staring at the floor from time to time. Then he said, "Heather, how come you broke your leg?" I replied, "I don't know, Bradley, that's just what happens." Bradley gently reached out and touched my leg in the splint. He began to say, "But, you still have your leg, right?" I said, "Yes, Bradley, I still have my leg. I will be fine. My leg will stop being broken soon." As Bradley looked on intensely, he fiddled with a toy in his hand and said, "Oh, I thought that your leg was broken right off." I laughed and said, "You're silly, Bradley." Bradley smiled and said, "I guess I have to go now before I'm late for school. I will see you later." I replied, "Okay." Once Bradley realized that my leg was still attached to the rest of me, he went off to school a relieved and much wiser little boy.

# Chapter 3

# The Rodding Surgery Begins

The summer after kindergarten, rodding surgery was scheduled for my legs for the end of August (see chapter 18 for details about this procedure). This surgery had never been done in Thunder Bay. When it became clear that it was in my best interest to have this surgery, my parents assumed that the procedure would be done at the Hospital for Sick Children in Toronto. My mother was concerned about how long we would have to stay in Toronto. The three other children at home, the costs of staying in another city, plus the daily household expenses, when Dad was the sole breadwinner, were a lot to be concerned about. Mom knew that it was important for her to be with me in Toronto, but leaving my sisters and brother at home was tearing her apart. Then our family doctor told Mom and Dad about a young orthopedic surgeon, Dr. Jack Remus, who had just opened his practice in Thunder Bay. He had studied under the same doctor in Toronto who was scheduled to do my surgery. Because he had a special interest in OI, he had learned the rodding procedure, but he had never performed this procedure on his own. My parents made an appointment to talk to him about doing the procedure in Thunder Bay.

During the meeting, Dr. Remus explained, "Not everyone with OI needs intramedullary (IM) rods. Children who do not fracture often and have straight bones do not need rods. Rodding is recommended for children who have curved bones or who repeatedly break a long bone, like Heather does."

Mom asked, "Can you explain exactly what the rodding surgery is?"

Dr. Remus answered, "Rodding surgery is the placement of a metallic device called a rod or nail into the internal cavity (medullary canal) of a long bone. This is major surgery, and the pros and cons should be carefully evaluated. Rodding is most often used to treat children with moderate to severe osteogenesis imperfecta. In teens and adults, it is usually reserved for difficult fractures that are not healing."

Dad asked, "Will you do both legs at once?"

Dr. Remus replied, "We will perform an initial round of surgery, consisting of four procedures done over four weeks. Starting the rodding procedure as soon as possible is important to allow the bones to grow straight, give them more stability, and prevent them from fracturing. The goal is to place the rods in both the upper (femur) and lower (tibia) bones in her legs, leaving the joints at the knee, ankle, and hip free to move. After one section of each leg is done, the leg will be placed in a cast."

Mom spoke up, "How long will she have to have the cast on?" Dr. Remus said, "Casts or splints to support the rodded limb are often needed for about four weeks after surgery, since healing time for OI bone is usually normal. Some children with OI do heal faster. Casting following femoral surgery is more difficult. Therefore hip spica casts and A-frame casts (a bilateral long leg cast with a connecting bar that prevents rotation) is an option. A *spica* extends from the ribs down the affected leg. This is required if fixation in the bone needs external support to heal. I can only decide during the surgery whether this heavy, postoperative immobilization is necessary. Whenever possible, most surgeons experienced with OI prefer to avoid spica casts, choosing an above-the-knee splint or lightweight plaster or fiberglass splints instead. Because people with OI face frequent periods in a cast due to surgery or fractures, steps should be taken to prevent immobilization osteoporosis. A guiding principle is to immobilize the broken or rodded bone with lightweight material for the shortest possible time. An above-the-knee cast or splint is used following tibia surgery. The knee may be bent so that the child can sit in a wheelchair or stroller."

After that initial meeting, my parents felt confident in Dr. Remus's ability to perform the surgery, which was scheduled for that fall. Dr. Remus became my orthopedic surgeon that day and remains so to this day. I had the first of four operations. Because the surgery was a fairly new procedure, my parents were asked whether they would allow my surgery to be filmed and allow the instructors to use it in the local university's nursing program.

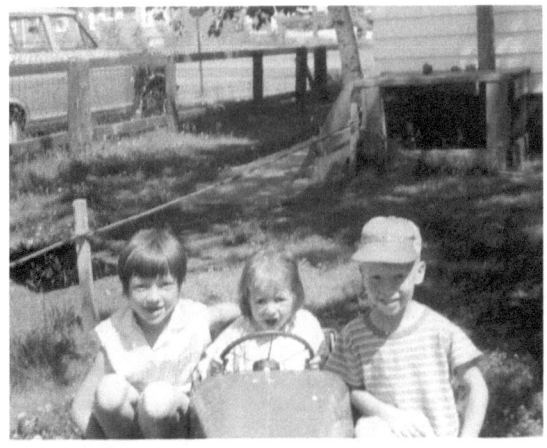

*L. to R. Carol, Heather (in go-cart), Clifford, summer of 1968*

My siblings and I took every opportunity to play together as long as I was feeling fine. So the time I was about to spend in the hospital away from them was hard on all of us. Carol, Clifford, and I often played in the backyard with our go-cart or on our swing set. I think we were all a bit anxious about the day for me to be admitted in to the hospital, which was fast approaching.

Even though I was only five years old when I had the surgery, the memory of that day remains vivid. It was a beautiful, warm, lazy summer afternoon. I had my favorite pink dress on. Mom always made sure we were dressed appropriately. Carol had come with me to ride my tricycle around the neighborhood before leaving for the hospital. I remember the warm breeze blowing through our hair. Carol and I were chatting up a storm and picking dandelions and pin cherries along the way. We were having so much fun, without a care in the world. Even though I knew that I was going to the hospital that day to be admitted for surgery the next day, I was completely unaware of the journey that lay ahead of me. I remember Mom calling us from the doorway of our house; we were just down the road a bit picking pin cherries off a tree on the boulevard when we heard her calls. Years later my Mom said to me, "I hated to call you back that day. The sun was shining so bright, without a cloud in the sky. You always enjoyed the outdoors so much. My heart was breaking with thoughts of uncertainty as your father and I struggled over whether we were making the right decision."

When I went into the hospital, my sisters and brother were not allowed to visit me because children were not allowed on the pediatric ward. The hospital staff was adamant about enforcing this strict rule, and they were not about to make any exceptions. This stubbornness made the surgery even harder on my siblings and me. They needed to know that I was going to be fine, but excluding them made it much more difficult for all of us to endure the experience. My parents begged the hospital staff to allow my siblings to visit. This

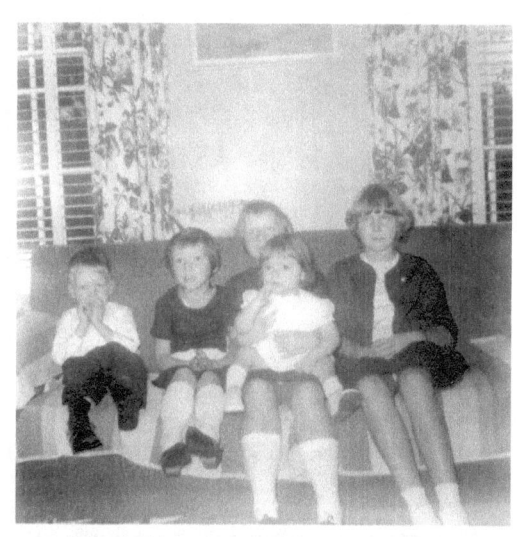

*L. to R. Clifford, Carol, Sheila (holding Heather), friend Anita Peterson. The day Heather went to the hospital to begin surgery.*

was not a simple case of day surgery or a stay of a couple of days in the hospital. This rodding surgery was serious business and meant a long recovery time. There was no support available to us to lessen the burden. My first stay in the hospital lasted three months, and the only contact I had with my sisters and brother was through a fifth-floor window and the occasional time Dad would sneak them up to the fifth floor. Dad used to bring them to the parking lot at the hospital, and Mom would wheel my stretcher to the window in the playroom overlooking the parking lot. From there, we could see each other and wave. As time went on, Dad would sometimes bring them up to the ward on the elevator while Mom and I would wait nearby. They would jump off for a little while, and we would hug each other and talk for a few minutes, always looking around to make sure no one was coming. I don't really know how my sisters and brother managed to deal so well with everything that was going on. We've never really talked about it, not even to this day. I suppose that I had so much to deal with myself that I never had the time or the energy to think about what it was like for them.

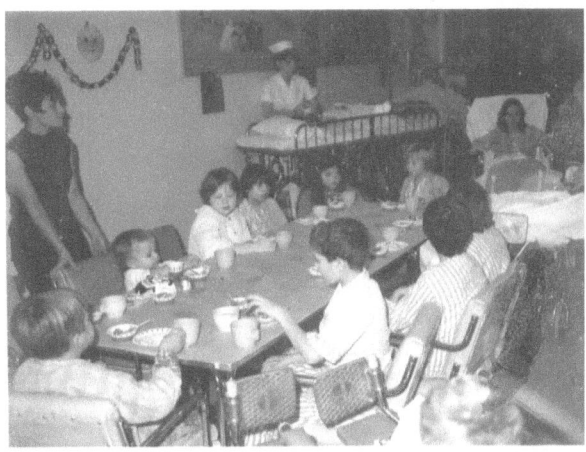

*Heather on stretcher after surgery in hospital playroom, September 1968*

One day when Mom came to the hospital, she said, "When I was getting ready today to come and visit you, Carol became very upset." Carol had said to Mom, "Why does Heather have to be in the hospital all the time? You spend so much time there, but we never get to go see her." Mom explained to Carol, "Honey, I know that you would like to go see her, but there is really nothing mommy can do. The hospital does not allow children to visit. I'm very sorry that it makes you so sad—it makes all of us sad. We have to wait just a bit longer, and then Heather can come home."

My brother was the second youngest in our family, and I think that he really missed not having Mom at home much. She was spending so much time at the hospital that I think he really suffered from the lack of attention. I remember that Mom started having him meet her downtown at Eaton's every Friday after school, which was only a block down the road from the hospital. She would spend the afternoon with me; after the dinner trays were served she would run down the road to Eaton's to meet Clifford. Dad dropped him off, and the two of them would window-shop, have dinner, buy a toy, and spend some time together. Then Dad would pick him up and the two of them would go home. Mom would come back to the hospital until late in the evening. My oldest sister, Sheila, was about fourteen years old when the rodding surgeries started. Mom really relied on her to help at home while she was spending so much time with me at the hospital. Sheila did most of the cooking, cleaning, and shopping when Mom was not able to and Dad was at work. I think that it made her grow up too fast. I always looked at her more like a second mother than a sister.

Sheila and John began to date when she was thirteen. I was only two years old when Sheila met John; she would have been eleven then. John always felt more like a brother to me. He was my buddy when I was growing up. We spent many hours playing games and cards. I still have a little troll doll that he gave me when I was a young child.

When I think about all the time that I was in the hospital, I remember the endless hours spent looking out the window of my hospital room and wondering when I was going to begin living my life. There were so many hours and days when Mom would push me on a stretcher around the pediatric ward just for something to do. She says that she wore a hole in the floor on "Peds." The doctor waited a week between each operation for me to regain my strength before he rodded the other section of the leg. After four weeks, the surgeries were finished. I was in a body cast from my rib cage to my toes. A stick connecting one ankle to the other was plastered into the cast to separate my legs and hold the bones in the correct position during the healing process.

People did their best to keep me occupied. I remember the special kindness of Gwen, my mother's dear friend, who collected games, books, puzzles, and anything else that she thought would interest me. She wrapped each one individually and told my Mom to bring me one gift every day. This went on for months. What a wonderful idea it was! This became something that I looked forward to each day, and I would wait patiently to find out what I would get to open, stimulating my mind and making some of my toughest days a little easier to bear.

I know that situations similar to the one my family faced can really make or break a family, but despite the challenges and the obstacles, we survived and endured. We had issues like every other family, and we kids got on each other's nerves from time to time, but I know that even though we've never really talked about the thoughts and feelings that we had during those years, our bond remains solid.

We knew right from the start that I would be in the hospital when the new school year began. My parents decided that once I was feeling better and was settled back at home, I would resume my education. My parents had made arrangements through the board of education for a private teacher, Mrs. Ditchfield, to come to our home to teach me. Should I go back in the hospital for any length of time, she would continue teaching me at the hospital. No one was sure how long it would take to rehabilitate me enough so I could return to regular public school. Once I was settled back home, grade 1 would begin.

# Chapter 4

## *Home from the Hospital*

I was in that body cast for nine months, unable to sit or bend my knees and ankles. Over those months, the cast was replaced every three weeks for hygienic purposes and to give the doctor a chance to make sure that my bones were healing properly. I was in the hospital for three months. I got home from the hospital on December 1, 1968, just in time for Christmas. Mom and Dad rented a hospital bed, along with everything else that we needed during my recovery. Our living room became a makeshift hospital. For the next twelve months, Mom slept on the couch near my bed. She cooked, cleaned, baked, and took care of Dad and us. She held Christmas gatherings, celebrated Easter, and organized Valentine's Day, Halloween, and birthday parties; and she never skipped a beat or complained. I remember those months as some of the happiest times in my life. Even though there was a long recovery and more physical pain ahead, I remember more than anything else that we were together as a family. I had my siblings to play with, we celebrated every family event, and we were happy. Life continued, with me in my hospital bed in the middle of the living room.

People thought that we lived in a big house, but the shape of that roof made the house seem bigger than it actually was inside. All the bedrooms were on the second floor, and that's why the living room became my bedroom. This was the perfect place for me to recover:

There were windows all around the room, so I never felt shut in. I could see people going by and birds flocking to the many bird feeders that Dad had put in the trees in the yard. I had sunshine all day long. At Christmas, the fireplace crackled with a warm fire, and the mantel was decorated with stockings for our pets and us.

That first Christmas home from my very long hospital stay was a lot of fun. Our home had very high ceilings, so we always had a freshly cut tree at least six feet tall in the living room. Once Dad put the lights on the tree, we kids would cover it with all the decorations we could find. I was in my hospital bed, so I could not actually help decorate the tree that year, but I had fun pulling decorations out of the boxes and handing them to my siblings. Last to go on the tree was the tinsel. In those days, everyone threw shiny gold or silver tinsel over the branches to give a sparkly look, like snow, I guess. Then we would all stand back and admire our glorious masterpiece. I was so excited to have this big, beautiful glimmering tree in my "bedroom."

On Christmas Eve my parents invited another couple over for a visit, and that couple brought a friend who was visiting during the holidays. Years later Mom told me that the fellow who came over with their friends cried after he left because he couldn't understand how my parents could be so happy and celebrate Christmas when they had a child who was "so bad off." In my parents' eyes, life was just unfolding the way it was meant to, and we were all genuinely happy. Later that Christmas Eve, after all the company had gone and everyone else had gone to bed, Mom and I settled down for the evening, me in my hospital bed in the corner of the living room and Mom on the couch, which was now her bed. The fireplace crackled as we watched the snowflakes falling to the ground. As I looked out the window, I saw Santa walking down the back lane. I yelled, "Mom! Mom! Look, there's Santa!" She got up and looked out the window with me. Then she said, "Oh, it *is* Santa. You'd better get to sleep because he's going to wait until you're asleep to come here." When I got older, Mom and I reminisced about that night. "Santa" turned out to be a neighbor who was returning home from a Christmas party. There could not have been a more magical moment for any child. That was my fondest Christmas memory ever.

We headed into the New Year of January 1969, and I was set to start grade 1 with Mrs. Ditchfield. She would follow the curriculum that the other students were following at my public school. I remember the first day Mrs. Ditchfield came to our home; she said, "Very nice to meet you, Heather. We have lots to cover because you have been off the past four months, so we better not waste any time. I also expect you to keep up with all the homework that I give you. When I come back the next time, you will need to have everything done." I felt a lump in my throat and thought. 'This is really going to be tough. I have no choice but to have all my homework done because I'm the only one in the class.'

I don't remember exactly what Mrs. Ditchfield looked like, but she was a small woman with dark hair. She was married, with children of her own. She had been teaching, children who were sick and unable to attend regular school for many years for the board of education. She came three times a week for four hours at a time. It was up to me to make sure I did the assignments she left for me in between. Eventually I settled into a routine and began enjoying what I was learning. Mom would make sure on the days I had school that the house was quiet for me to learn.

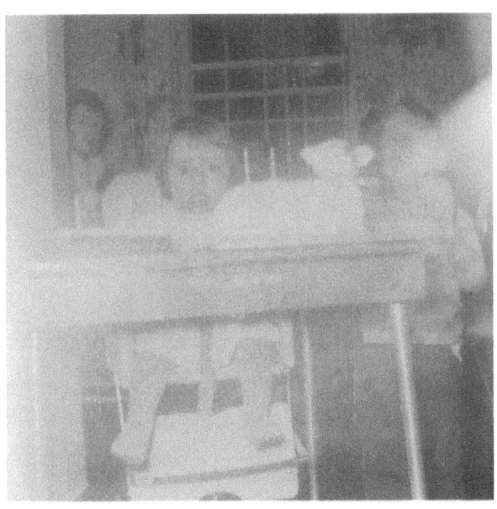

*Lamb cake Nanny always made for us. L. to R. Carol, Heather, and Clifford. This picture was taken back when Heather turned two years old.*

When Valentine's Day rolled around, Mom asked us kids, "Should we have a party and invite all of your friends?" Of course we yelled, "Yeah, let's have a party!" Clifford and I each invited a few of our friends; Sheila and Carol were getting too old to want to do things like that. Sheila was busy with high school, her part-time job at the corner store across the street from our house, and her boyfriend, John. Mom said, "Maybe we can ask Nanny to make a heart-shaped cake for us." Nanny always made us cakes in different shapes for different occasions. (I remember pictures of the lamb-shaped cakes she made for each of us when we celebrated our birthdays.) We kids made cutout hearts, and Mom hung them over the kitchen table. We had a red tablecloth and of course our heart-shaped cake. A good time was had by all. Of course, we had to celebrate St. Patrick's Day as well—that's Mom's birthday. I remember we had pancakes that morning for breakfast, and Carol said, "Wait, Mom!" She ran to the cupboard, got a candle, and stuck it in Mom's pancake. Then she turned to her and said, "Happy birthday, Mom."

Nanny and Grandpa always came to our house for Easter dinner. Nanny like to attend church on a regular basis, so she would take Sheila, Carol, and Clifford with her to church while Mom stayed home with me and got dinner ready. Dad and Grandpa would stay home with Mom and I. They were not the type to attend church, except if Mom or Nanny made them.

May was just around the corner; it would mark the ninth month that I had been in my body cast. Even though we went to the hospital every three weeks to have the cast changed and a new one put on, now would be the first time that the cast would be permanently removed. So we thought.

I had hated having the cast changed each time because it was always so painful. To this day I cannot stand the sound of the cast saw. As the saw cut the cast, it would heat up. Despite the fact that I was always told that the saw would not cut my skin, I could feel my tender skin burn, especially the incision. Also during the time it took to quickly start wrapping the new cast back on, my legs were unsupported, which created a great deal of pain. When the day finally came to remove the cast once and for all, no one was looking more forward to it than me.

Neither the doctor nor the staff had prepared my parents for the long road to recovery. None of us knew exactly what to expect when the cast was removed. Mom and I anxiously looked on as the top half of the cast was removed. Mom later told me, "I took one look at your legs lying limp and lifeless in the lower half of the cast. I was horrified, and it was all I could do to stay calm in front of you. I told the nurse that I needed to go over some things with her in the other room. My body was trembling, and I felt as though I was going to pass out. I was in a state of complete shock, and as I entered the other room with the nurse I fell apart. "What have I done by allowing this surgery? Look at her legs—this was meant to help her, not make a mess out of them like that! I have ruined her life."

The nurse immediately contacted the doctor, who explained to my mother that everything was going to be fine. My legs were skinny and seemed lifeless because they were not completely healed yet, and they would need more time in the cast, as well as extensive therapy to regain lost muscle. Mom told me, "The nurse made me a cup of tea and let me pull myself together for a while before I went back in to the room with you."

After talking with Dr. Remus, Mom felt reassured that she and Dad had made the right choice after all. Now that the body cast had been cut in half, the top half of the cast could be taken off when we wanted to wash my legs or to simply let them get some air. Since my legs needed more healing time, I was to leave my legs in the bottom half of the cast and just remove the top from time to time. A tenser bandage was wrapped around the entire body cast to keep it together, so when we wanted to remove the top half of the cast, we would just unwrap the tenser bandage. I cannot tell you how nice it was to be able to scratch my legs after nine months. Mom would gently wash my legs with a face cloth, and the dead skin would peel off, as well as the scabs from the stitches that ran down the front of my legs from my knee to my ankle and down the sides of each leg from the top of my legs to my knee. Not a pretty sight.

That spring my Aunt Greta had phoned and told my mom, "I'm going to send the kids bunny rabbits as a gift for passing school." Mom said, "You are going to send them what?" Aunt Greta was a really easy-going, fun-loving person. She knew that we kids loved animals. So she figured that this would be a great joke, as well as fun for us kids. My parents never really took her seriously and thought that she was just joking. Well, around the middle of May we received a really big delivery in a giant box. We kids were all excited when we found out it was from our Aunt Greta. Mom and Dad opened the box that said "Live animal, handle with care!" What do you know? Out jumped four huge white bunny rabbits. I remember us kids laughing and screaming as we tried to catch the big bunnies to hold: one for each of us, just as she had promised. Mom got on the phone and called Aunt Greta and said, "Greta! I thought you were just joking about the bunnies!"

Greta burst into laughter and said, "Do the kids like them?"

Mom said, "Yes, the kids are going crazy over them! You do realize that we cannot keep four big bunnies in the city?" Aunt Greta just laughed again.

We had to keep them in the basement in a homemade pen for a week until we found a farm interested in taking them. We kids had a blast with them. Of course, I was unable to care for them, so that part was left to my siblings and Mom. We enjoyed them very much until we brought them to the farm in the country that welcomed them among all the other farm animals. None of us forgot that experience. My Aunt Greta really liked a good joke.

June was fast approaching, and I spent the rest of July and August getting used to having the top half of the cast off. Mom would remove the top half of the cast and put me out in the sun to play for a while each nice day and then replace the top, lay me on my stomach, and remove the bottom half. When August rolled around I had a beautiful tan on my legs. I remember all the nurses saying, "How did you get such a beautiful tan? Your legs look so good."

That summer we stayed close to home since I was still in the body cast and unable to sit up. We spent a lot of time outside playing in the yard and just enjoying the nice weather. Dad had made me a cart with wheels low to the ground, just like a mechanic's cart, that would accommodate my legs, which were separated by the stick. I was able to lie on my stomach and push myself around with my hands.

I remember when my parents, my sister Carol, and I went downtown in our station wagon one sunny Saturday afternoon. Because I was still in the full body cast, I was lying on my stomach in the back of the station wagon. Dad, Carol, and I stayed in the car because I was unable to sit, which made getting around difficult for me, while Mom went into the store to pick up what we needed. As we waited and chatted, a group of elderly women noticed me as they walked past our car. They turned, came back to our vehicle, cupped their hands against the window, and stared at me while pointing and speaking to each other in their own language.

We were shocked by this vulgar and incredibly thoughtless behavior. When Mom came back, we told her what had happened. She wanted to know why Dad hadn't said anything to them. I guess that he was so stunned by their actions, he could not respond to them. We couldn't understand how people could be so hurtful and rude. Not until I started writing this book did the memory of that incident came back to me. I spoke to Carol and asked if she remembered it, and she did. We were both very young, yet that incident made a tremendous impression on both of us. We were fortunate that because our parents loved us and accepted us unconditionally, we were able to hold our heads high and rise above the ugliness in this world.

At the end of that August, I was scheduled to begin therapy four hours a day, five days a week. So that meant I would start grade 2 with Mrs. Ditchfield at home instead of returning to my public school at Black Bay.

# Chapter 5

## *Rehabilitation*

In September 1969, fall arrived, and a new school year was ready to begin. I started the long road to recovery. We were not sure how long therapy would be needed—only time would tell. What we did know for sure was that the road ahead was not going to be easy. I continued to use the lower half of the cast, keeping it in place by wrapping it with tensor bandages. I no longer needed the top half of the cast, which was removed, but I had become weak from being in the cast for so long. I always said that I remained in the body cast for nine months but technically much longer than that, because after the first nine months I remained in the lower half of the cast to support my legs until they were strong enough for it to be permanently removed. That would turn out to be well over a year. During this time, Dr. Remus kept a close eye on my recovery, usually checking in every month. Before I began therapy, Dr. Remus told Mom and me, "Physical therapy is required for most children with OI after rodding surgery. Some physicians prescribe physical therapy during the recovery period to keep up muscle strength in the limbs not affected by the surgery. Other times, physical therapy, sometimes beginning in the swimming pool, is employed after the cast is removed to help the individual regain strength."

When I started therapy, I was so weak that the therapist very gently would lift me from the bottom half of the cast because it was so painful for me to move my legs. Sitting up for the first time in months was a task in itself. The therapist would lay me on a canvas stretcher that was hooked to chains bolted into the ceiling and gently lower me into the water. This procedure continued for many months until I was strong enough to move my legs and sit up by myself. I remember the first time Mom put me on the floor to sit up for a while and play, about six or seven months into therapy. At the time, we had a Pekingese named Sandy. He had quite a cranky personality, and he let Mom know that he did not think I should be sitting on the floor. Because he had never seen me do that; to him it was wrong. He barked and walked around me, all the while looking at me and then at Mom, trying to tell her to pick me up.

Therapy continued every day for the rest of that year and into the next year. I was home-schooled by Mrs. Ditchfield during the mornings, three days a week for about four hours each session, through grades 2 and 3. Mrs. Ditchfield was very strict. There were days when I was so tired from the grueling therapy, I just didn't want to learn anything, much less do homework. Mrs. Ditchfield never wavered, though, and when she assigned homework, she expected me to do it. I remember complaining to my parents, saying, "The teacher expects me to have so many assignments done, I cannot keep up." So my parents asked her, "Mrs. Ditchfield, don't you think that you should give her a break, she's been through so much?" Mrs. Ditchfield responded, "My job is to teach Heather and make sure that she keeps up with the required standards expected for the grade that she's in. I realize that she's been through rough times, but she can do this. She's a bright little girl." My parents explained the importance of keeping up with my grades and said that I just needed to do the best I could. Like all kids do, I tried to get out of having to do an assignment. When I think back to those days, I'm glad that Mrs. Ditchfield was such a great teacher and had such high expectations of me. She became more than just my teacher; over the years, she became friends with my whole family.

Afternoons were reserved for therapy. Dad dropped Mom and me off at St. Joseph's General Hospital rehab about 1:00 PM after lunch and then picked us up at the end of each session around 5:00 PM

Each new school year, I was "placed" in the grade and classroom at my public school, even though I wasn't actually there. I kept in close touch with my classmates so that I wouldn't feel out of place when I returned to

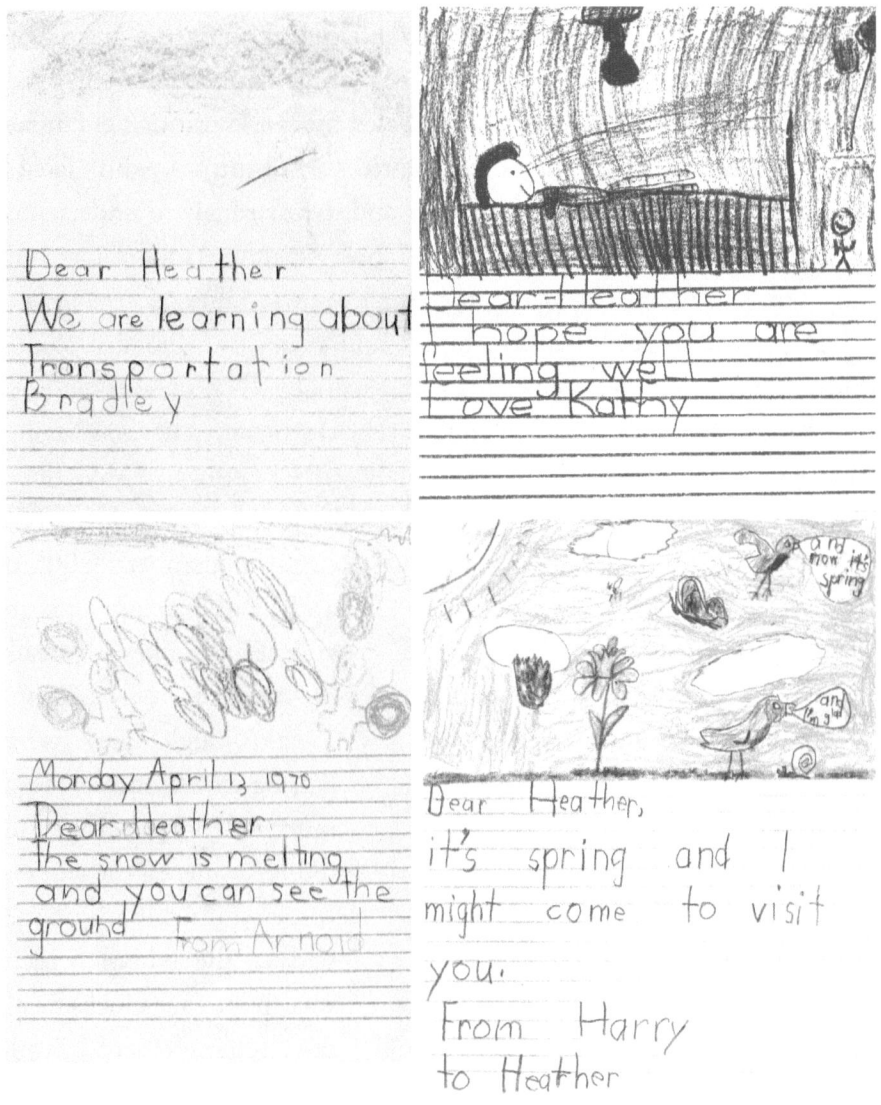

school. They all knew that I was being taught privately. I remember the great kindness of my teachers, who had their students write to me during those years. The letters were meant to make all of us feel connected and part of one another's lives. The children let me know what was going on in their lives, and it helped the teachers explain how I was doing and why I wasn't at school with them. Each year, they compiled a scrapbook of those letters. Reading through those scrapbooks reminded me that I belonged. Every once in awhile when I'm cleaning things up at home I come across those old scrapbooks. They bring back a flood of good memories. Each one of those letters revealed the world through children's eyes: for example, what they each wanted for Christmas, who "liked" whom, why so-and-so got a detention, and their struggle to understand why I couldn't be in class with them. Those scrapbooks are a precious keepsake. The friends I had met the year I went to kindergarten, before my surgery, like Carol, Cathy, Bradley, and Harry, continued to come down to my house on a regular basis after school and on the weekends to play. Mom would take me to my public school when my class was having a party for special occasions, such as Halloween, Christmas, or Valentine's Day, so that I would feel like I was still part of the class.

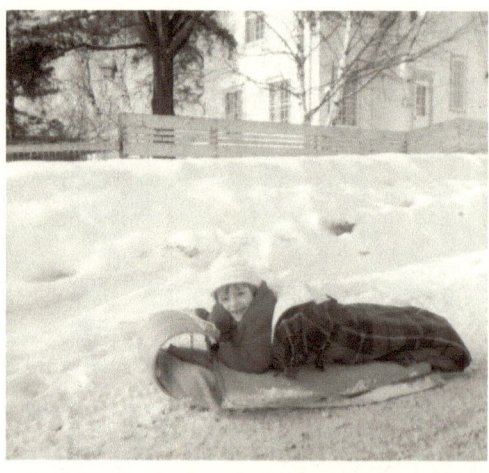

*Heather on sleigh with full body cast on after surgery, in front of family home*

I remember Clifford and Carol going out to collect for Halloween treats for me when I was laid up. Even though they were getting to be too old to go out for Halloween, they still did it for me. In the winter, Mom would pull me on the sled to the school, which was about four blocks from our home. When I wore the body cast, I would lie on my stomach and Mom would wrap a blanket around my cast, and off we would go. That's how we went out for walks in the winter as well, so that I could get some fresh air and play in the snow.

Both my sisters were old enough to go downtown by themselves on a Saturday afternoon. I remember that Carol always bought me a huge round lollipop with her allowance. Sheila had her own spending money from working at the corner store. She spoiled me, too. My siblings really sacrificed a great deal. Some parents try to shield their children from unpleasant situations, but in our case, we had no choice but to experience it together.

By the end of grade 2, I had finally become strong enough for the body cast to be removed permanently. This had been a very slow and gradual process, as I mentioned earlier. Simply learning to sit up again after laying flat on my back or stomach for so long took me months to conquer.

You're probably wondering if I still experienced other fractures during that time. The answer is yes, occasionally—not as often or as frequently as before the surgery, but little fractures would still happen. Although my legs were in the body cast, which was up to my ribcage, for over a year before it came off completely, every inch of me was fragile, so that meant that the rest of me was vulnerable. Despite everything, I did quite well during that time.

We spent the summer once again enjoying the warm weather and doing some camping as a family. Now that the cast was no longer on and I was sitting up and moving about quite well, we were able to be a bit more active. When we went to see Dr. Remus just before summer started he explained, "Braces may be used after the removal of the cast to provide added support for standing and walking."

Mom said, "What is the purpose of the brace?"

Dr. Remus replied, "A brace is worn to protect the limb, as the patient becomes more active. Children who have had surgery on their tibias often require a period of post-operative bracing." So that summer

I was booked to be fitted for a brace so that once I returned to therapy in the fall I would learn to walk with the braces and use crutches.

In the fall of 1970, I returned to therapy to begin learning how to walk using the braces and crutches. I hated the braces; they were heavy, awkward, and uncomfortable. I continued to attend therapy for four hours each day. Part of that time I was in the pool doing exercises to help build strength, and the rest I spent in the gym. In the gym were a small set of walking bars that I used while getting the hang of walking with the braces. As time went on I gradually advanced to walking with the help of crutches instead of the bars. I was doing quite well, but I needed someone close by to make sure I did not fall.

My parents decided that I would complete grade 3 with Mrs. Ditchfield at home in the mornings, as we had been doing. The goal was to return to regular public school for grade 4. Continuing with home schooling seemed logical as long as I needed to attend therapy. The rest of that year played out pretty much like the previous one: school at home in the mornings and therapy in the afternoons. By the end of the school year, I was getting around quite well, so Dr. Remus and my parents decided that it was safe to allow me to return to public school and to cut back on the therapy, as long as I continued to exercise and practice walking at home.

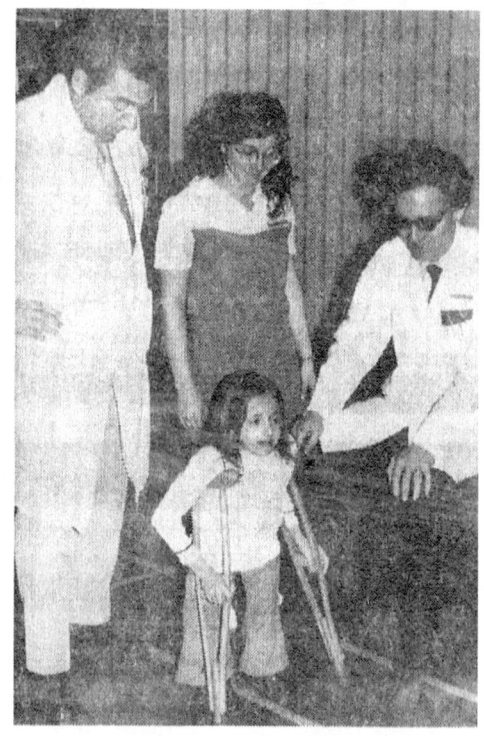

*Heather learning to walk with braces and crutches at therapy*

## Chapter 6

## *My Return to Public School*

Finally in September 1971, I went back to regular school for the first time since kindergarten. I attended grade 4 classes in the morning and spent three afternoons a week in therapy.

I was so happy to be attending public school again. Despite the fact that I liked Mrs. Ditchfield and we had shared many good times during my home schooling, I had longed to be back at school with my friends. I received my first wheelchair to start grade 4 that year. Being tiny is one of the traits of having OI, so even though I was seven years old, I was much smaller than the average child, and the wheelchair was much too large for me. I don't ever remember seeing smaller wheelchairs for children back then. Although my new wheelchair was large I was still delighted to be able to get around.

That year we lost our little dog Sandy to an eye disease. A year before, he had lost his left eye, and this year the disease affected his right eye. We had no choice but to put him down. Dad felt that having a pet was important for us and even more important for me, because I was more housebound than my siblings. So he got me a

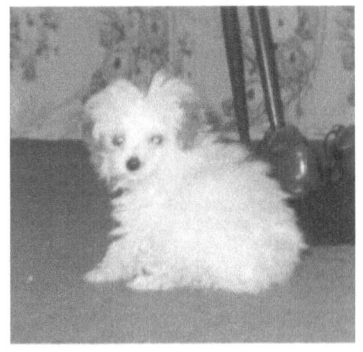

*Muffin – family pet*

little teacup poodle named Muffin. She was apricot colored and small enough to ride in the wheelchair beside me. I took her everywhere I went. She was a source of great comfort to me.

Dad made me a gym at home so that I could continue to exercise and get stronger. Dad took all the measurements and had a welder make the equipment my size. He turned our basement into a mini-gym with tiny walking bars and weights; everything that we used at therapy in the hospital was duplicated and set up for me at home. When you walked into our basement, it looked like you were walking into a professional gym, only pint-sized. After that, I could keep up with exercising as much as I wanted without having to go to therapy at the hospital.

That first year back to public school was better than I had anticipated. I met my two best friends, Lori and Jeanette. We started spending a great deal of time together in school and outside of school. Jeanette and Lori were the same age as me but a lot taller. They were both average height for seven-year-olds, but I was only about two feet tall. Lori and I had dark brown, shoulder-length hair. Jeanette had short brown hair. Lori had two sisters and a brother, and they lived only a few blocks from my house. Jeanette lived a few blocks from my house as well. She had three sisters. Over the years my parents became friends with both Lori and Jeanette's parents. Our families often planned camping trips together during the summer.

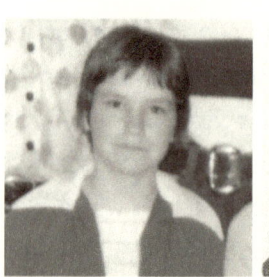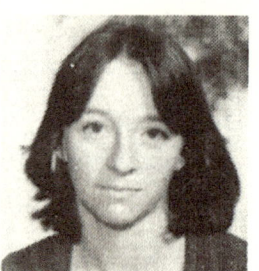

*L. to R. Jeannette and Lori, Grade 4*

By the end of that school year I no longer needed as much therapy because I had the mini gym at home. When the following fall rolled around, I began to prepare for grade 5. This was the first time in four years that I would not need to attend therapy. I felt as though I was beginning to lead a somewhat normal life once again, except for the ongoing fractures, which were an expected part of OI.

One day I was playing on the living room floor with a beach ball. I was trying to lean back on the ball, but it rolled away. I fell flat on the floor and twisted my left arm behind me. Naturally, my arm broke quite badly, and I couldn't move because I was in so much pain. Every time I tried to move or get up off the floor I could hear and feel the bones cracking and rubbing together. I cannot even begin to describe the pain. I felt as though I were separating from my body, like an out-of-body experience. I imagine that's the body's way of dealing with traumatic shock. I remember Dad saying, "Don't try to get up, just stay still. I will be right back."

Mom ran to the phone. I recall hearing her say, "This is Margaret Anderson. Heather has had a fall and broken her arm. I will be bringing her in to the ER. Please call Dr. Remus." In those days if you needed your doctor, the nurses would put a call out an emergency call to alert him.

In a split second, Dad ran out to the garage and made a makeshift splint out of map tubing that he cut in half. He held the homemade splint and said to me, "Slip this under your arm so that I can lift you off the floor and take you to the ER." I was starting to feel cold from the shock; I just wanted to get to the ER so they could make the pain stop. I remember saying, "All right, just don't move my arm too much."

When we arrived at the ER, we learned that Dr. Remus had called in and said he would be arriving soon. The nurses left that splint on my arm until I was taken to the OR. The next day at Dad's work, the staff nurse approached him and handed him the splint. She said, "Eric, I'm so sorry to hear that your daughter broke her arm again. I work at the hospital part-time, and I was working the OR last night when you brought her in. All of us in the OR were so impressed with your ingenuity that we saved the splint and wanted to give it back to you." My dad, not a man of many words, just said, "Thank you, I appreciate your thoughtfulness." He smiled as he walked away. Dad was very touched by her comments.

This kind of incident may be shocking to others who are unaware of OI, but they had become a normal part of our lives. Many doctors and nurses are completely unaware of the extent of OI. Whenever I've been hospitalized or taken to the ER for treatment, they usually take the opportunity to ask me about OI. I've even had other doctors who are not involved in my case ask me whether their residents could examine me and ask a few questions. I really don't mind explaining my condition and sharing my experiences with them. Reading about OI in a medical book is not quite the same as getting the chance to meet someone who lives with the condition every single day.

Most of the kids at school understood that they had to be very careful around me. Hitting, punching, and playing rough were off limits. All kids, including me, sometimes forgot that rule in the heat of the moment. I remember one day at recess, my friends and I were goofing around on the school grounds, and I grabbed Carol by the arm. She began to run after Cathy, and in a flash, I heard my arm snap. Oh, yes, the familiar sound and the rush of pain once again flooded me. I screamed out,

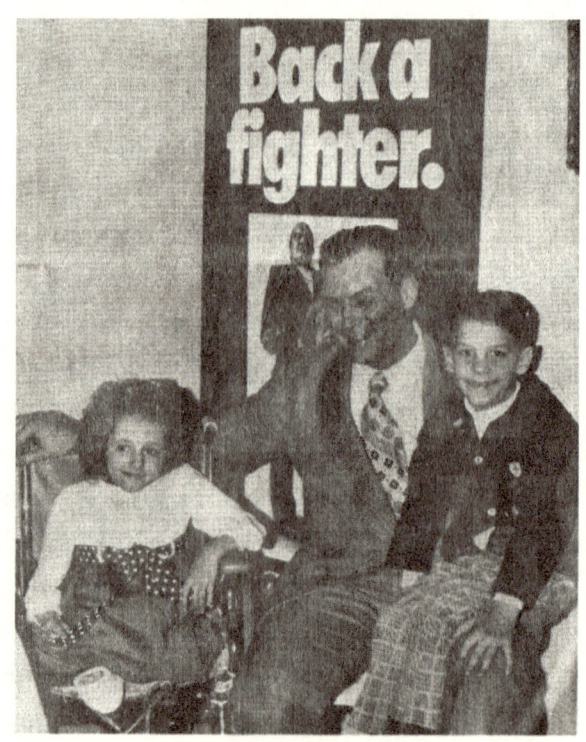

*Easter Seals Campaign*

"I broke my arm." The girls both stopped in their tracks with looks of horror on their little faces. Before long, all three of us were crying. The teacher noticed the commotion and came over to us. The teacher called the principal, and I remember him telling me, "I don't think you broke your arm, you probably just sprained it." I said, "My arm is broken, I know how that feels. Please call my mom." Mom also understood that my arm was broken, so off to the hospital we went.

Most people have difficulty understanding the extent of my fragility. When I used to get really severe episodes of hiccups, Mom would have to hold my back because my skeletal structure was so weak and it would hurt so much. Because most people just didn't believe that I could fracture something that easily, they always doubted me, and that was always the hard part for me. Mom used to tell family and friends, "Don't call me during school hours, because when I hear the phone ring while Heather is at school my heart stops. I think that the school might be phoning to tell me that Heather got hurt." Sure enough, Mom received that inevitable call all too often over the years. I don't know where my parents got the strength to meet each challenge that happened while I was growing up or how they were able to stay so calm in emergencies. I was blessed with wonderful parents.

Mom would get the dreaded call the next time when I was in grade 6. During recess, the wheelchair suddenly tipped when my friends and I were playing, and I fell out. My friend Carol had accidently put her foot on the foot pedal of the wheelchair, which caused the wheelchair to tip. She was very upset, but it wasn't her fault. Off to the hospital I went again, but this time I lucked out—I had a few sprains and two chipped front teeth. We were all hoping that I would be able to recover quickly because I had been chosen that year by the local Easter Seals program to represent our area.

The Easter Seals Campaign selected one boy and one girl to represent the organization based on how much each had improved and how far they had come in their recovery. The girls were called Tammy and the boys Timmy. So that year I was the Tammy for the local Easter Seals Campaign, called "Back a Fighter." The Timmy and Tammy were honorary guests at the campaign dinner, as well as at other functions throughout that year. I was really honored to have been chosen that year. I would remember the experience my entire life.

That year we lost Muffin due to complications when we had her spayed. My heart was broken along with the whole family's. The vet who performed the surgery felt so bad that this had happened to my pet that he wanted to get me another. Within a few months, the newest member of the family arrived—another apricot teacup poodle we named him Tuffy. For a while all was right in my world again. Tuffy soon accompanied me everywhere I went.

By the time I had finished grade 7, my parents realized that I no longer needed my exercise equipment. Dad came to me and said, "Heather, you really don't need your mini gym anymore, so let's donated it to other kids that might have a need for it." I said I thought that would be a wonderful idea. Mom said, "How about donating it to the George Jeffrey Children's Foundation for children with disabilities?" Both Dad and I agreed that would be the best place. Many children made use of that homemade mini gym over the years and benefitted from it as much as I did.

The summer before grade 8 I lost my beloved Tuffy. We never knew exactly what had happened to him, but we were fairly certain he had been stolen. Our yard was completely fenced in. One evening around 10:30 PM Mom let him out before bedtime. Not more than fifteen minutes went by before Mom went to the door to call him. He was nowhere to be found. Dad searched the neighborhood most of that night. In the weeks prior to his disappearance there had been talk on the news of people stealing purebreds from people's yards. For weeks we had everyone who knew us searching. Signs went up, and the humane society was notified. We never again saw our Tuffy. Once again my heart was broken. I wanted to wait a while before getting any more pets because we were not having much luck. I think we all needed time to heal.

In the five years after my return to public school, at least a couple of times a year I was back in the hospital having surgery or having a section of my leg re-rodded. As a child grows, the rod becomes too small for the bone, and chances increase that the leg will start to bow where there is no rod. I remained very tiny in size and did not grow much, but the rods needed to be replaced in sections of my legs during my public school days. Usually I remained in hospital for only a few weeks and was able to return to school with a cast on the repaired section of leg. Sometimes after a period of time the body might begin to reject the rod if it changed position and it would need to be replaced for that reason alone. Of course, there were the never-ending fractures, which also sometimes required surgery.

During one of my many hospital stays, I helped to paint a mural on a wall on the pediatric ward. Because I spent so much time in and out of the hospital, I developed a real bond with the nurses and staff. I was mature for my age, and I enjoyed the company of adults as much as I enjoyed being with children my age. The staff had begun painting murals on the walls throughout the ward, and they asked me if I would like to help paint a mural on the wall. I replied, "Yes, I would love to help." So later in the evenings, once visiting hours were over, a few other nurses and I would paint children hand-in-hand in a circle on the main mural across from the elevators. The idea came from the hit song "Black and White" by Three Dog Night. I was so proud that I could contribute to that painting, especially because of the powerful meaning behind the song. That hospital is now a long term-recovery facility and hospice. The paintings that once graced the walls were painted over long ago, but the memories of those days will stay with me forever.

—

Sheila and John married on August 2, 1975. Carol and I were both in the wedding party. Using my braces and crutches, I was able to walk down the aisle. The ring bearer was my cousin Brenda's son, only five years old at the time, yet he was already taller than me. In the fall I would start grade 8.

Just after Sheila and John's wedding, my Uncle Kenny and Aunt Pat moved to British Columbia. Two of their children, Brenda and Roy, were the only ones staying behind. They were both married with families of their own and choose to stay in Thunder Bay. We were sad to see the other family members go, as our families spent a great deal of time together.

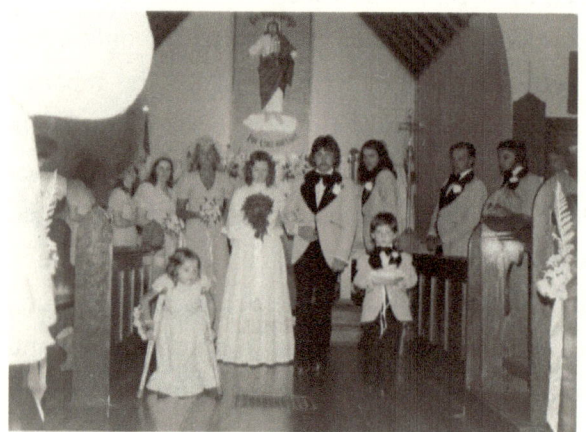

*Heather walking down the aisle at Sheila's wedding, 1975*

We also got a call that year that my Aunt Greta had passed away. She never came back to town for a visit after she moved but she kept in contact now and again by phone. She loved playing jokes on people. We always remember her for the time she sent the big bunnies.

As grade 8 neared its end—the year seemed to go by so quickly—the time came to start thinking of high school. In the late 1970s, not many schools wanted me as one of their students. My parents and I knew that I would not be able to attend the high school in our district because that school had stairs everywhere. We narrowed our choices down to two others. Although they were not wheelchair accessible, we felt that we could work around their obstacles. Near the end of grade 8, Lori and her family moved to an area of the city that happened to be close to one of the two high schools on my list. That meant that we might go to the same school. I talked to her about my situation, and she convinced me to choose her high school. She promised that she would help me do whatever was necessary to get around the school. Her parents were in full agreement with our plan. My parents spoke to the administrator of Lori's school and said, "Heather will need to make a choice between this high school and one other in the city that we feel will work for her." The administrator replied, "Are you sure this is the best school for her? We're really not equipped for the disabled." So my parents spoke to the administrator of the second school on my list, and he stated, "Maybe it would be better for her to attend the first school on your list, as we're really not prepared for a disabled student." Ultimately, my parents had to tell the administrators at my school of choice rather firmly that I would be attending their school in the fall.

# Chapter 7

## *Entering High School*

At the beginning of my grade 9 school year, Lori and I met with the school counselor. He helped us plan our schedules, making sure that we were both in the same classes so that Lori could help me. If we were taking different subjects, which meant being in different classes, Lori would be allowed to leave her class five minutes early to take me to my next class. To this day I'm not sure how Lori found the energy or the strength to fulfill the task. This was a physically demanding job for anyone to do every day. She was probably no more than a small-framed five foot five inches. She was not overly athletic, but she kept active and never strayed away from helping others. A lot of kids at school asked if she and I were sisters. I guess they just assumed that since she was always there to help me, we must be related.

The high school had two flights of stairs up and one set that went into the basement. We had to make sure that my subjects upstairs or downstairs were grouped together. That way, I could avoid going up and down the stairs more than twice each day. Lori carried me, and another person from our class was assigned to bring the wheelchair up or down the stairs. Lori and the other students took on a tremendous responsibility each day in order to help me out. They continued to help day in and day out from grade 9 through grade 13.

Lori helped me work things out until I became more comfortable with my surroundings and began to meet new friends. Then my new friends would help at different times, so the burden for Lori decreased. Nevertheless, she was always there whenever I needed her help. I really owe Lori and everyone else who helped me during those years a great deal of gratitude. They made it possible for me to get an education. How can I ever thank so many people who gave so much of themselves? I cannot express how much they meant to me then; they will always hold a special place in my heart. I believe that people come into our lives when we need them the most. They are angels sent from God.

In the 1970s, schools were not only unaccommodating on the inside, they were also unaccommodating outside. The only action that the local board of education took to accommodate my needs was to install a ramp outside one of the school doors. The problem was the ramp was in a tow-away zone. Because the bus wasn't equipped to carry passengers with disabilities, I couldn't ride it, so I again went to school in a taxi provided and paid for by the board of education, as I had in public school. The driver wasn't supposed to park near the ramp when he brought me to school or picked me up. The police gave him a lot of parking tickets over the years!

The taxi company did not want to be held responsible if something happened to me, and once again, Mom was there to help out. The taxi company made her ride back and forth with me each day. Yes, Mom rode that taxi every single school day for five years. She always joked that she went to high school for five years but never graduated. Mom laughs when she recalls an incident that she will never forget. She said, "Each morning when we dropped you off at school the taxi driver would ask me if I would mind if he stopped at the carwash nearby before bring me home. Of course I didn't mind, so I always said that's fine. This ritual continued for several months, and I never gave a second thought about what this must look like to someone else. And one day the young man that was taking the money at the carwash looked at me with the most disgusted look, as if to say 'Lady, do you ride around with taxi drivers every day?' I told the driver, and the both of us got a good laugh out of that one."

Since my high school had no other students with disabilities, everyone needed a period of adjusting. For the first few months, I'd hear my name called over the PA system asking me to report to the nurse's station. So off I would go from class to the nurse's station, and the nurse would say, "Heather, is everything going well? Do you need time to rest?" I remember thinking to myself, 'Do I need time to rest? What is this, kindergarten?' I would reply that everything was fine and return to my class. This went on for several months, until it became a joke with my friends in class. One of the kids would say, "Isn't it time for Heather to go to the nurse's station?" We would all laugh. Finally I told my mom. She could not believe what was happening. She contacted the school and told them that she appreciated their concern, but I was fine and would not need a rest during classes.

My grandpa passed away that year at the age of eighty-five. He had been diagnosed with cancer. This was the first death of a family member who was close to us kids. We all took it hard. Nanny was ten years younger than Grandpa, so she was still very active. She continued to live in the same house, which was close to ours, so we were able to see a great deal of each other, like before. Jeanette and I often walked to her house to play cribbage.

Jeannette and I still spent a great deal of time together, even though we were no longer at the same school. We often spent the weekends together at Sheila and John's place. We loved spending time there, especially after they had their first baby. Amanda was born on May 31, 1977, my first niece and the first grandchild for my parents. We all adored her. Both Sheila and John were very close to my parents and us kids. (As I said before, John had been around almost all my life. He seemed like a second brother to me.) My parents loved having Mandy around. Mom looked after her when Sheila went back to work at Lakehead University, where she'd worked since she graduated from high school.

Carol had been working at the grain elevators since she got out of high school. Dad had helped her get the job, and Clifford was hoping to get a job there as well. He was not as happy in high school as I was. He wanted to just get it over with and find a job. When Dad got him on at the elevators, he was much more content working than going to school.

The summer before I started grade 10, my Aunt Betty came to town with her daughter Lois Ann for a visit. This was the first time we had seen them since they moved. I was very young when they moved, so now that I was older I had the chance to really get to know her. Aunt Betty and I got along great during the month that she stayed with us. We started writing to each other on a regular basis once she left. I really enjoyed getting to know her.

When I was in grade 10, a few of my friends and I went sledding one weekend evening. My parents never stopped me from doing activities that were within reason as long as I was fully aware of the consequences, although Mom said, "I let you participate in as much as you could, but my heart was always in my throat." That evening was a beautiful winter night; big snowflakes were falling down. We were only going to go a few blocks from my house and have some fun on a small hill in the park. I got on one of the sleds, and someone pulled me. The evening was going well, and we were all having fun. At about ten o'clock we all thought we had better head home. Jeanette said, "Heather, I will pull you home on the sled." When we were about one block from my home, the sled hit a patch of ice and slid in front of Jeanette. When she lifted her leg, her boot clipped my elbow. I felt a strange feeling in my arm, and something told me to look down. When I did, I could see my left arm dragging. At that moment I felt a surge of pain and realized that I had fractured my arm. I remember screaming, "My arm is broken." Jeanette stopped, took off her mitts, and put them under my arm to try and support it. When we got to my house, Jeanette ran inside crying and told my Mom. Dad was home watching Saturday night hockey, like he did every Saturday night. We piled into Dad's truck to the hospital once again. When I was given pain medication at the ER, we were all able to take a moment to gather ourselves. We then realized that Jeanette had frozen her baby finger because she took her mitts off. The nurse took a look at her finger and said it wasn't badly frozen and would recover. I was whisked off to the OR to have a steel rod placed in my arm. I spent a couple of days in the hospital and returned back to school with a cast on. It happened to be close to Christmas exams. My doctor asked me if I wanted a note from him so I would be allowed to write mine later when I was feeling better. I didn't want to prolong studying so I went ahead as planned, despite how uncomfortable I felt.

I've endured so many injuries doing simple activities that I can't even recall how many or which bones I've fractured, but it's certainly more than a hundred. Fractures have become a normal part of my journey. For people living with OI, most fractures occur before puberty.

High school was shaping up to be a really great time for me. Despite all the issues that we had to deal with and overcome, it was proving to be a happy and memorable time.

# Chapter 8

## *My Senior Years in High School*

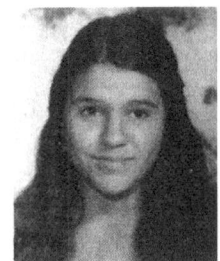

*Rina*

I made some great friends during my last years of high school, including a new friend named Rina. We met in grade 11 because we sat beside each other in computer class. Rina was a pretty, dark-haired Italian girl with a bubbly, outgoing personality. We bonded right off the bat and began spending a great deal of time hanging out together at school.

The school year had started out great, and everything went smoothly until an incident happened midway through the year. I had taken a class that year called law, which consisted of getting to know the basics of the criminal justice system. A couple of weeks during the year we would go to the local courthouse and sit in on cases being tried. Our assignment would be to write an essay on those cases. We also conducted mock cases in the classroom. Everyone really enjoyed this class. One particular day, a friend from law class who usually helped me was away, so she made arrangements with another girl in our class to take over for her. The girl had helped out in the past with the wheelchair, but she had never carried me down the stairs. We all felt comfortable with her doing this for the first time. After she picked me up, she stepped on a piece of paper on the second staircase landing and began to lose her footing. We never went right down the stairs, but we did stumble around. I think she may even have hit the wall before we fell.

Students and teachers in the classrooms nearby heard all the commotion, and the teachers immediately came running over to help us. They realized the seriousness of the situation and began to block the area off from students who would soon be getting out of class. I'll never forget the look on my law teacher's face. We had just come out of his class. He ran over to offer help, but I knew that I was hurt badly. I couldn't move, so he stayed there and held my head up until the ambulance arrived. The girl who had been carrying me was unhurt, but she was shaken and very upset. News traveled fast throughout the school, and everyone who knew me was trying to get past the teachers' blockade to make sure that I was okay.

I remember Lori telling me later: "I was at my locker deciding what books I needed for my next class when a girl with her locker near me said, 'You know your friend in the wheelchair, Heather?' and I said 'Yes, what about her?' The girl said, 'Well, she just fell down the stairs and everyone's crowded around. I think they're waiting for the ambulance.' What she was saying didn't click with me right away, and I turned and looked at her and said, 'What did you just say?' The girl repeated, 'Heather—she just fell down the stairs.' I dropped my books, left my locker open, and started running toward the stairs. I was not sure which staircase she meant, so I yelled back to her as I was running, 'What staircase?' She yelled back, 'The middle one.' I was so afraid; my heart was pounding. I could not get there fast enough. When I finally got there, the teachers pushed me back, saying, 'You can't go up there.' I pushed past and made my way to the top. Do you remember seeing me?"

I said, "Yes, I heard you asking me if I was hurt bad, and then the teachers pulled you back and made you go down to the bottom of the stairs."

Lori said, "I was so upset, I just left school and went home to tell my mom."

This was a really traumatic event for the whole school. My friends told me that the next morning, the principal announced that I was fine, but I would stay in the hospital. I had small fractures in my right arm and left knee. Every inch of me hurt from suffering so many strained muscles.

When I returned to school a few weeks later, I felt like a movie star. Everyone, even students I didn't know, would say, "Hi, Heather. I'm glad to see you back." Some would say, "How are you feeling now? Let me sign the cast on your arm." That was quite a time, but we all survived. My mom phoned the girl who had been carrying me. She told her, "This was an accident. I don't want you to feel responsible because this is not your fault, and no one blames you. I am grateful that you had been trying to help Heather." I think the girl had a rough time getting over the fall. No one wants to have something like that happen, but that's just life. We never really know what's in store for us.

For the most part, my high school teachers were really great people. I admired and respected most of them, but the one exception was my grade 11 science teacher. He and I just never saw eye to eye on anything. I think that it was simply a personality conflict. He never thought that I actually had done my homework myself, and he implied more than once that my friends did the work for me. I remember him saying at the beginning of many classes, "Heather, did you really complete this assignment or did your friends do it for you?" I replied, "Yes, I did it myself. Why would you say that?" The teacher would reply, "Your friends seem to do everything for you." I remember that the entire class would get involved; everyone would shout at the teacher. "Why do you ask Heather that all the time? She does her homework. We don't do it for her." This really was quite insulting and embarrassing. I think that he felt that I should have been at some other high school—any other high school than the high school where he was teaching. I was the first student with a disability to attend that particular high school. He made life so difficult for me that I told my parents I wanted to be transferred out of his class. Mom spoke to the principal about the situation. She said, "Just because Heather uses a wheelchair does not make her incapable of thinking." The principal said, "I understand why you're upset, Mrs. Anderson, but it won't do Heather any good to change classes so late in the year." I stayed in that science class for the rest of that year, but I never took another class with him. I wonder whether he ever changed his attitude.

I experienced a similar incident only one other time in high school. During grade 12, I wanted to take a theater arts course, and the vice principal said, "Perhaps, Heather, you should reconsider. There is a lot of physical activity involved when a person is acting. If you had a scene where you might have to walk across the stage and shake hands with someone, you wouldn't be able to do that." My answer was, "Then I would wheel across the stage and shake hands with someone." Naturally I took the class and had a great deal of fun. I got a good grade for my efforts.

I made a lot of good friends during those high school years, and we share some wonderful memories. I often think about all those loyal friends, who accepted me and helped to make everyday life at school easier for me. I felt lucky that the generation I grew up with was so accepting and caring. A group of eight to ten friends remained my steadfast companions throughout high school.

Since I was uncertain of what I wanted to do with my life, I decided after I graduated from grade 12 to return and finish grade 13, which was an optional year if you wished to go on to university. Grade 13 has since been intergraded into the four-year curriculum and no longer exists in Canada.

In September 1980, Sheila, John, and Mandy moved to Calgary due to John's work. We were all devastated. The move was hard on all of us because we spent so much time together. I remember crying for days after they left. Sheila was eight months pregnant with their second child, and Carol was pregnant with her first child. Both were due around the same time. My parents decided that Mom and I would go out to Calgary to be with Sheila for the birth, and Dad and Clifford would stay home to be with Carol. Mom was hoping that we would have time to get back before Carol had her baby. I took a couple of weeks off school, and Mom and I took the train. Flights were expensive at the time, and the train offered a much better deal. We thought it would be kind of fun to experience the train.

Sheila was having a cesarean the morning that we were to arrive. John and Mandy picked us up, and we all went straight to the hospital. Adam entered the world on October 31, 1980. He was beautiful. The day before we were scheduled to come home, Dad called to tell us Carol had a beautiful baby girl. Mom was disappointed that we had not arrived home in time. Leaving Mandy and Adam was hard, but we were also anxious to get home to see Carol's little one. When Dad phoned us in Calgary to tell us all about Amie, Sheila really wished she was coming back home with us. I remember I cried the whole way home. Dad picked us up at the train station, and we went straight to see Carol. Amie was born November 12, 1980, twelve days after Adam. She was beautiful. Mom took care of Amie when Carol returned to work. Carol worked at the elevators like Dad, except she did shift work. Amie often spent the night and the next morning at our house so Carol could get some sleep, depending on what shifts her partner was working. This gave us a great opportunity to spend a lot of time with Amie right from birth.

When grade 13 ended I still had no idea what direction to go with my life. I had taken many summer art classes during high school, so I was leaning toward fine arts. I began to think that maybe I should consider going to university.

# Chapter 9

## *Learning to Drive*

When I was eighteen, the local board of education started the first driver's education program for drivers with disabilities. I was among the first group of students to participate in the program and receive my driving license. Most of my friends had been driving for quite some time, so this program was a wonderful opportunity for me to learn to drive, as other students did. Driving gave me a freedom that I had never known before, because it was the only thing that I could do by myself.

My driver's education course started in the fall and ran throughout the winter months. The instructor would pick me up in the vehicle that had been equipped with hand controls. I remember the weather being snowy on the nights my driving lessons were scheduled. That experience helped me become very comfortable with winter driving. Shortly after I received my license I bought a vehicle. People sometimes think that having a disability entitles me to all kinds of government perks. This is not true. Government assistance helped to pay for the hand controls and other devices that would help me gain my independence, but I paid for my car myself. I did all kinds of stuff when I was growing up to make money. Dad used to make birdhouses for me out of leftover lumber from jobs he had done, and I would paint and sell them. I also sold Regal for many years. From these odd jobs, I had saved enough for a down payment. The subsequent low monthly payments stretched out over four years.

After I got my car and had it equipped with hand controls, I would drive for hours. I'd turn on the car radio, listen to some music, and enjoy my new freedom. The destination didn't matter. When I was driving along the highway in that car, I was just like everyone else. Once I got settled into that car I was fine on my own. No one else needed to be with me; nothing else gave me such a feeling of complete independence. Eventually I realized that I needed to figure out a way to get in and out of the car without assistance. I looked into the available assistive devices and found

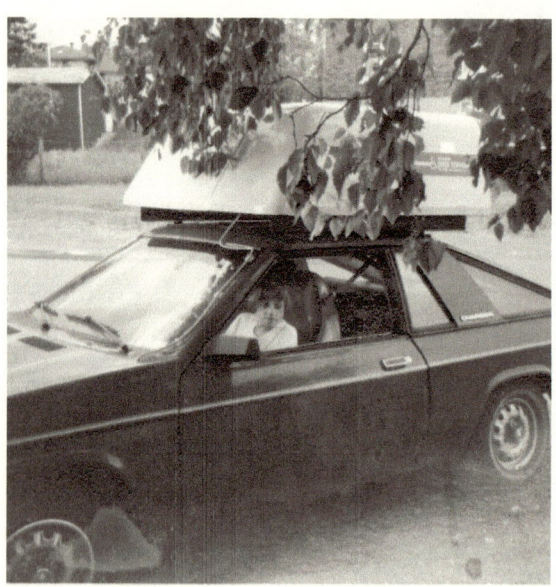

*Heather driving her car with wheelchair lift on top*

a wheelchair lift that fit on the roof of the car. I could operate the remote control from inside the car. After I opened the driver's door, I would slide into the car from my wheelchair, and then all I had to do was press a control to open the lift on top of the car. A hook on a chain would come down that I would place under the seat of my wheelchair, and then I'd press the control. As the lift raised the chair to be even with the car roof, the wheelchair would turn sideways and slide into the roof topper. Once the latch door closed, I would shut the car door and drive off. When I wanted to get out all I had to do was press the control to lower the chair. Then I'd get into my chair from the car seat and go about my business.

Because I was so small, I had to sit on a big pillow folded over in order to be high enough to see over the steering wheel. Using hand controls meant that I did not have to worry about how far from the gas and brake pedal my feet were because I only needed to use my hands. Dad was the first one to test out the hand controls after they were installed. He wanted to make sure that everything was working properly. I do recall Dad saying, "Once you get the hang of how things work, I kind of like driving with the hand controls and not having to use my feet."

I remember people being so impressed and pleased that I was able to drive, no one more so than my Uncle Kenny. My aunt and uncle loved children. After they moved to British Columbia, he and my aunt adopted two more children. Uncle Kenny came for a visit and brought one of the girls with him to meet us all. My aunt was unable to get off work at the time. The other adopted daughter stayed home to be with my aunt. Uncle Kenny said to Mom, "I can't believe that girl—nothing stops her! She's just amazing."

Nanny was another person who was ecstatic that I was driving. She used to say to me, "Heather, you don't drive at night when it's dark, do you?" I would say, "Yes, Nanny, I do." Then she would turn to Mom and say, "Margaret! You don't let her drive at night, do you?" Mom would say, "Of course she does." Mom and I always got a kick out of that. Nanny was a funny lady.

One beautiful sunny Saturday afternoon, I picked up Nanny. We were going to go to the grocery store to pick up a few items. I pulled up in the wheelchair spot. Before we had a chance to get out of the car, this older fellow started walking toward my open window. He said, "You young punks have no respect for anything. Can you not see that spot is reserved for people in wheelchairs? Damn you kids, you're all smart asses." Before I had time to say anything he turned and walked away, grumbling under his breath. Nanny was very hard of hearing, and she said, "What's he saying, Heather? Why is he yelling at you? Hey, mister, what are you yelling at my granddaughter for?"

I was so shocked and taken back by what the man was saying that I was not sure what to say or do. Nanny could not hear what was going on, but she knew he was yelling at me. The fellow had not noticed that my license plate displayed the wheelchair symbol, which meant that I was a designated user for that spot. (These days, a sticker placed on your dashboard indicates if you are able to legally use a wheelchair spot.) It was nice that the fellow was looking out for others, but maybe he just went a little bit overboard. I get mad myself when I see people taking those spots when they don't need to, but you have to be careful about jumping to conclusions. Sometimes a person may look fine physically and still have a right to use the spot. We have to remember why those spots are designated. They are not there because the disabled want to be treated specially but because for the physically challenged, pushing a wheelchair across a parking lot or walking, especially in the winter, can be very difficult.

I always say it would be wonderful to not need a wheelchair spot. Rather than misusing the designated spots, able-bodied people should be grateful they don't need one and remind themselves that one day they may actually need that spot. Then they will realize the difference.

# Chapter 10

## *First Two Years After High School*

Even though I knew I wanted to eventually go to university or college, I still wanted to work a bit to get a feel for the working world and make sure that whatever career I choose would be right for me. Entering the workforce was not easy for me. I applied to many jobs; after what seemed like a ton of interviews I still had no luck. Since I had no real formal training of any kind at that point in my life, there were not a lot of options. Being small and in the wheelchair meant that not all jobs were suitable for me. Most places were not considered accessible, unlike today. I was unable to work at fast food places or any of the kind of jobs that the average student would take due to my condition. This made my search for employment just a little tougher than most kids'. Most of my friends from high school had already settled into jobs or continued with further education.

The lack of accessibility in offices and other local venues is still one of my biggest issues. When applying for a job, most people don't give a second thought as to how accessible the building might be for someone who is physically challenged. They also don't have to think about how they're going to get somewhere or how they're going to get in once they get there. I always have to assess where I'm going, how I'm going to get there, and how I'm going to get in. Simple tasks like paying bills or going to appointments are major challenges. Even though I drive, the fact that

I still need some physical assistance because of my size has always been a hindrance. Being small—and I mean really small—has presented many challenges. I guess that all little people can relate to my dilemma. We just don't live in a world that easily accommodates people who are only three feet tall. One drawback to being small is that I'm not exactly the strongest person in the world. And although using my wheelchair makes navigating daily life easier, I have found the most inaccessible places are doctors' and dentists' offices and churches. These places aren't easily accessible to people who use wheelchairs or who can't climb stairs.

Most people don't think much about such barriers because they're not personally faced with them on a regular basis. Wouldn't it be great if I could wake up, even for just a few days or a week, and go about my day in a barrier-free world? Wow, that would be like a dream come true! An even better dream would be to go shopping in any store and find adult clothes and shoes in my size that don't have cartoon decals on them. I would love to go shopping for whatever style shoes I want. Have you ever gone shopping for shoes that look nice and match your outfit … but in a child's size nine? Yes, that's right, a child's size nine. I think that my nieces and nephew had outgrown that size by the time they were five years old, if not before. My dream is to pick out any style that I want … in my size. I continually shop for shoes, no matter what city or store I'm in, because if I find shoes that suit my style, I buy them. Remember, my shoes never wear out, so most of them look brand new—forever!

I had not received a letter from my Aunt Betty in quite some time, and we all were concerned about what had happened. Mom contacted Lois Ann, who informed us that her mother had been diagnosed with Alzheimer's disease. That was the reason the for the letters stopping. Lois Ann had not been aware that my Aunt Betty and I wrote back and forth. Because she was trying to cope with the diagnosis, she had not yet informed us. For a long time after, I really missed those letters.

That year, Mom, Carol, Amie, and I decided to go to Calgary for a visit. Sheila and Carol had not yet seen each other's children, except in pictures. That trip would go down in history, a bit like a Chevy Chase movie, right from the moment we stepped on the plane. Lasagna was being served for dinner on the flight. Oh, yes! Nice, sloppy red sauce. Amie was only a few years old. Of course, within the first few minutes Amie had totaled her napkin. So Mom

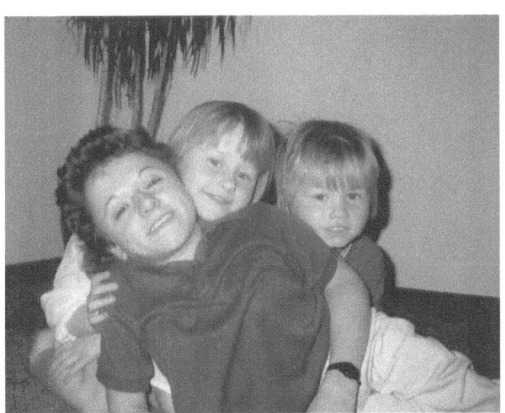

*L. to R. Heather, Mandy, and Adam in Calgary*

gave hers to Amie. At the end of the meal Mom forgot that she had given her napkin to Amie. Thinking that she still had it on her lap, she proceeded to wipe her hands on her pants—nice white pants. Carol and I could not stop laughing. That was just the beginning.

Because we had not been together in a while, we all wanted to have a good time and experience as much as we could while in Calgary. We would all pile into Sheila and John's car and off we would go to take in the beauty of the city. There were so many funny incidents. We seemed to end up fighting everywhere we went. The kids were all still very young; in the heat at the end of each day, they were *not* happy campers. Which in turn made tempers short. Later in the evening, we would reminisce and laugh about what went on each day. Mom seemed to end up with the two little ones hanging around her neck while the rest of us went off.

The one incident we all remember most of all was when we got to the hot springs at Banff. By the time we left the hot springs, both Adam and Amie were tired and screaming from the heat. Mom had one on each arm trying to calm them down. Amie kept yelling, "I want ju ju (juice)!" Adam just kept screaming. I remember Mom saying, "If you two don't stop, I'm going to run my head into that window." When our pictures were developed, we would go through them and say, "Oh, look, there we are fighting at the zoo! There we are fighting at the carnival!

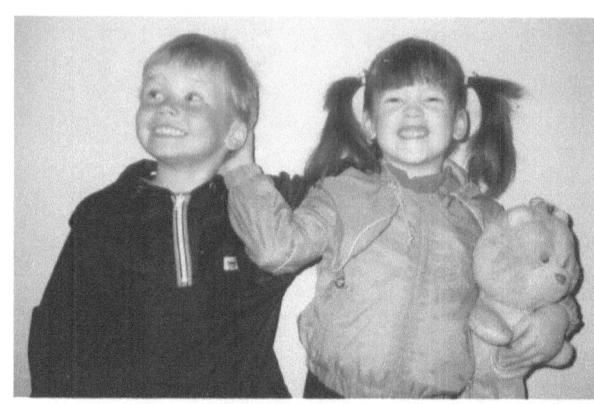

*L. to R. Adam and Amie (age 3)*

There we are fighting at Banff! There's Mom getting ready to slam her head into the window!" That trip was one of our craziest but most memorable times together.

When we got back home, I went back to my job search. As I said, I wanted to work for a while before really thinking about a career. So I went to the local youth employment office to find something suitable. I ended up doing fundraising for the George Jeffrey Children's Centre, the same center to which we had donated my mini gym. This job was not specifically for the disabled; anyone could apply. So I was hired, along with three others. The office was set up with booths for each of us to make phone calls from 9 to 4 to businesses for donations to the Centre. I didn't realize that Rina happened to be working for a company named Clarkson and Gordon. I had not seen Rina since high school; we lost track of each other for a few years. But her company was on my list to contact. We rekindled our friendship when she answered the company phone and recognized my voice. Rina said to me, "I'm getting married. Would you like to come to my wedding?"

I replied, "Yes, that would be nice."

Rina then said, "My fiancé John and I are going to build a house."

I asked her, "What part of town will you be in?"

She replied, "Down in Current River on Montclair Street." By sheer coincidence the house they were building was a block from my parents' home.

I said, "Rina that's the next block from my parents place, and I'm still living at home."

She laughed and said, "I guess we are going to be neighbors."

My job at the George Jefferies Children's Centre was a six-month contract, so it was not long before I was looking for work once again. My love of animals made me consider becoming a veterinarian, but that career would have created some challenges. I'm small in stature and not very strong physically, so I would have run into many roadblocks with that career. Besides, I would have wanted to take every patient home with me. I considered going to school in another community, but that decision would also have involved overcoming some major obstacles. I felt that whatever career I chose I would make it succeed. My next career option was to become a pharmacist. I wasn't sure if I wanted to be a pharmacist, so I enrolled in a student apprenticeship program called YES (Youth Employment Services). I had to pick a place where I might like to work, approach the business, and ask whether I could work there for six to twelve months. YES would pay me the minimum wage, and the business would have to commit to teaching me about the service it provided.

I was lucky enough to be accepted at the pharmacy in the hospital where I had spent so much of my childhood. I thought that would be the last place where I'd want to work for eight hours every day, but just the opposite happened. I felt quite at home working at the hospital because many people I knew from my time as a patient still worked there. The best change was that now I could go home at the end of each day!

On my first day of work, I pulled into the parking lot in my brand new car. I remember seeing a man standing by the loading dock. Stan worked in housekeeping, and he was unloading garbage off the loading deck. The sun was shining brightly, and a warm wind blew gently. As I got out of my car and into my wheelchair, I looked over at what he was doing. He smiled and said, "Beautiful day today." I smiled back and said, "Sure is." I recall thinking 'What a nice, polite, handsome young man.' The year went on, and we got to know each other and quickly became work friends. I was seventeen at the time, and Stan seemed to be much older than I. He was married, with one son. Many years would go by before we reconnected, but that story comes later.

I enjoyed my year at the pharmacy, and I learned many things—one of which was that I didn't want to be a pharmacist. Counting pills all day long just didn't do anything for me. I remained undecided about my career path. Unable to seek employment through the usual avenues, I went back to YES and asked them to sponsor me for another job. This time I thought I would try working in a nursing home. I really enjoyed being in a setting where I felt I could help other people. I guess after all those years when so many strangers helped me made me want to offer help in return. I enjoyed working at Grandview Lodge Nursing Home. My job was to assist the events coordinator, who organized all the events that took place in the nursing home. After six months, I decided that it was time for me to go back to school.

That September, two years after high school, I enrolled in the Fine Arts department at Lakehead University, hoping to rekindle my artistic ability. I was very creative as a child and loved to dabble in painting, drawing, and pottery. This seemed to be a logical place to start. By my second year in the program, I was feeling discontented, still searching for a direction that felt more comfortable.

Rina got married that summer of 1984 on June 9, and they moved into the neighborhood. As time went on, we began to spend more and more time together. We had many common interests, one being psychics and spirituality. Being young and inquisitive about the world and what was in store for us created a strong common ground that allowed us to begin to understand each other on a deeper level. Our hopes and dreams were big, and our journey in life was just beginning.

Before long Rina and John were expecting their first child. On November 21, 1985, their daughter was born. Having a family was important to them, and finding a career was important to me. I attended university and Rina cared for a newborn baby, and that was the start of our new lives. Those high school days now seemed far behind us, and ahead lay all our dreams.

# Chapter 11

## *First Major Job*

While I was working toward my degree in fine arts, I thought I would take the opportunity to explore one of my other interests: singing. So I took voice lessons as one of my electives. At the time I was also looking for a job. Early in December of that year the counselor who had been helping me look for a job told me about a position that she thought would be perfect. Lakehead University's Forestry Department was inter-

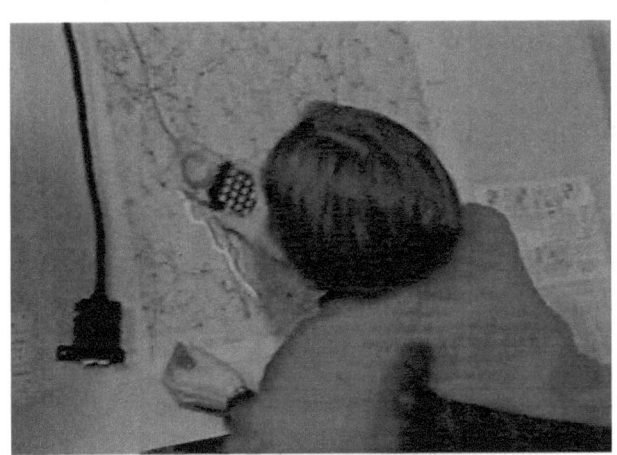

*Heather doing GIS mapping*

ested in training a person in geographical information systems (GIS) digitizing. The position required that the successful candidate have a working knowledge of computers, which I did not have, but the university was willing to fully train the right person. The counselor felt that I would be right for the job, so she encouraged me to apply. GIS was an up-

and-coming way of analyzing data on the computer using a computer program called Arc Info. Mining companies as well as the forest industries were beginning to use this technology. The component called digitizing took layers of information from a paper copy of a map to create data that could be used on the computer. A tablet, much like a drafting table, with a grid under it and a small device with crosshairs called a curser is used to trace over the map. The curser is attached to the tablet, which is then plugged into the computer. For example, when tracing contour lines from a map using the software program Arc/Info, the contour lines then appear on the computer screen. Important data can be attached to each contour line to enable the user to transform the data into a three-dimensional drawing on the computer screen. This could then be printed out using a plotter, which is basically a printer in a larger form. Through this method, the forestry industry was able to understand all kinds of information, such as burnt-out areas, replant areas, and tree types, like spruce, balsam, etcetera.

I remember the interview very clearly. The gentleman conducting the interview explained, "The successful candidate will be learning how to use the computer program called Arc/Info. Do you have any computer experience, Heather?"

I replied, "No, I do not, but I have an interest in learning."

The gentleman then said, "After you become comfortable operating the program, we will need you to take these paper copies of maps and input the required data from each map by digitizing them into the system. Then we can then use this data for several purposes."

I said, "Will there be someone to assist me as I learn the program?"

He said, "You will have all the help you need in order to become comfortable with the program before you begin with the maps." He then explained the equipment and their uses and outlined what they expected the trainee to learn. I was totally baffled by all of this information, but the possibilities held my interest. This was back in the days when computers were just starting to become common in the workplace.

The interview took place close to Christmas, and the interviewer mentioned that the successful candidate would be contacted early in January. We shook hands. I went home and never really gave it much more thought because I was certain that someone with more knowledge of computers would be hired. To my surprise, they called me during the last week of December to offer me the position. I was ecstatic! This would be my first full-time job since leaving high school. Plus I would be learning a trade in GIS digitizing. I decided to put my university classes on hold. For now life seemed to have a clearer direction for me.

I took to GIS digitizing like a duck to water. It opened up a whole new world to me, and I realized how much I enjoyed working with computers. I think my artistic ability helped me with the digitizing tasks, which required great patience and accuracy, very much like drawing or painting except that the medium was the computer. I enjoyed digitizing hardcopy maps and turning them into important and usable computer data.

In the days to follow I began to meet my coworkers one by one. As it turned out I would be working with five others who were directly involved in GIS, all men. I would be working closely under Grant, who was in charge of teaching me the program. Grant was in his twenties; he had a wonderfully kind and gentle personality. Then there was Joe. I would say he was in his early thirties. Joe and I never interacted much, and a year or so after I was hired he moved on to pursue other endeavors. Next was Peter. He was maybe in his early thirties as well and married with two children. He and I got along well, as I did with Grant. Before long we were very comfortable with each other and had become friends.

Ulf joined the team a few months after I started, coming from British Columbia. He was a forestry professor working toward his PhD. He was in his early thirties, recently divorced, and originally from Sweden. Since my dad was also from Sweden, this immediately gave us something in common. Ulf and I kind of started out on the wrong foot and did not exactly see eye to eye in the beginning. I'm not really sure why this happened; it was never anything major, just basically a misunderstanding that needed to be talked through. I remember talking to Peter about this. He said to me, "Heather, I want you and Ulf to sit down and work out whatever differences you two seem to have. I need a team that can work together." I agreed. Later that day Peter went and got Ulf and made him and me sit down and talk. By the end of that talk we had realized that we had no reason to not get along. From that day on Ulf and I ended up becoming the best of friends. Our friendship continued to grow.

Hans was the only team member who was a little older, perhaps in his fifties. On my first week on the job he came to talk to me and start to get to know me, I guess. I was twenty-one years old when I began my first full-time job, and I was a bit shy and insecure. Hans was European, with a somewhat direct and overbearing mannerism. I was not sure how to take this, so I came across as shy and withdrawn. Grant realized that this was happening, and I remember him telling me, "Heather, I told Hans to back off a bit and give you time to get comfortable with everyone." He laughed and said, "Hans can be a bit overbearing at times." After that I began to relax. Hans took a great interest in me. Beneath that gruff exterior was one of the kindest men I had ever met. Hans had three sons and a daughter. The first summer I worked for him, one of Hans' sons worked with me on one of the projects. I had a great summer, and I bonded with Hans and his entire family. In the years that followed we shared many wonderful times.

In my first year working there, a dog belonging to one of the housekeeping staff had a litter of puppies. I went home and told my family about the puppies. At the time, Clifford was trying to convince my mom that we should get a dog. Clifford and I were the only ones still living with our parents. One day when my sister Carol was at home visiting, I happened to mention the puppies. She said, "Let's go see what the puppies look like."

So Clifford, Carol, and I set off to see them. We took one look at them and fell in love. There was a white one and a black one. The white one was spoken for, so we gladly said, "We'll take the black one." That night we came home with our new puppy. Mom was not too thrilled, but she said, "He sure is sweet." Dad fell in love with him right away, like the rest of us. If my dad had his way,

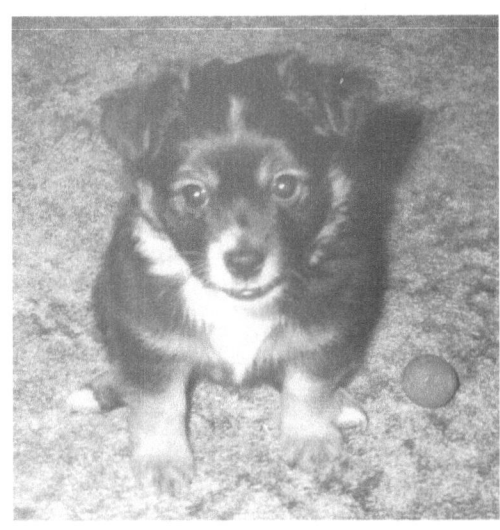

*Odie, first night home, 6 weeks old.*

we would have had more animals than Noah's Ark. We had him home about a week before we named him. Mom was the one that actually named him. She said, "How about we call him Odie, like the little dog in "Garfield"?" We all loved the name. So that day our pudgy little puppy was named Odie. He was part sheltie, with black, white, and tan coloring. He had the most beautiful white chest, just like a lion's mane. He settled into our home quickly, and before long he had won the hearts of everyone he came in contact with. He brought joy to everyone.

Dad had been having some difficulties with balance and vision that year. He used to come in the house from his workshop and say to Mom, "I don't know what's wrong with me. Lately I take my measurements and cut a board, and in the end I have a wrong measurement. I never used to make mistakes like that. My eyesight must be going." We were starting to get worried about him. All of us told him that he should go to the doctor and get things checked out. He would say, "Yeah, yeah, one of these days."

Sheila, John, Mandy, and Adam moved back home to Thunder Bay that year. We were all thrilled. Sheila had worked at the Lakehead

University prior to moving to Calgary. Now that she was back in town she looked for employment again. She began applying for jobs and ended up landing one back at Lakehead University in psychology, the same department she worked in before. Since I was also working there, we decided that we would ride together. I drove.

When my holidays rolled around after my first year of work, I wanted to go on a really nice vacation because this was my first really good job. My friend and I went on a cruise to the Caribbean and visited seven islands. What a fabulous experience, but there were some challenges on the ship. I'm sure that cruise ships are much more accommodating now. By far, air travel is the most accommodating mode of transportation for passengers with disabilities. I have flown alone a few times to visit friends, and the flights have been fine, as long as someone has been able to meet me at my destination.

I continued to train and work at the university over the next four years.

Two years after Sheila and John moved back to town, she gave birth to their third child. On September 12, 1986, Ashley was born. All of Sheila's children were born by cesarean section. Her due date was the week of Dad's birthday. So they picked the twelfth, Dad's birthday. Six years had gone by since Adam and Amie were born.

We were all delighted to have a little one around again. We all had so much fun with her. All of Sheila and John's children were blonde like Sheila, but Ashley was the only one with big bouncy curls.

Two years later on October 13, 1988, Carol gave birth to her second child, Rachel. She was the spitting image of Amie, with auburn hair and big brown eyes just like Carol. They both looked like little holly hobby dolls. Everyone was thrilled to have another little one around so soon after Ashley.

After my fifth year working in the GIS field I became more confident in my abilities. I was presented with the opportunity to offer my GIS skills as an independent contractor. The digitizing tablet, as

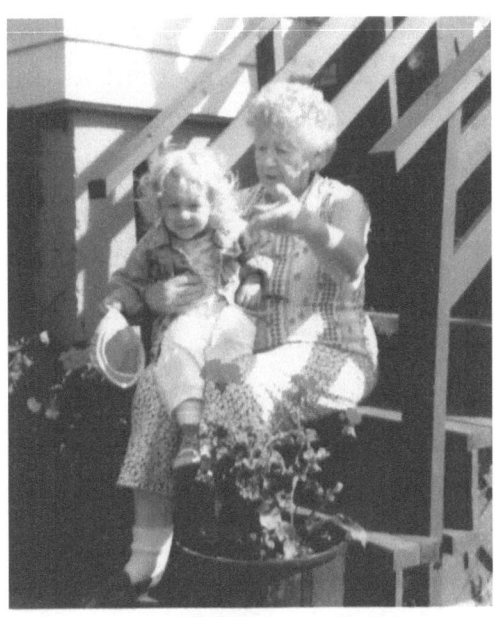

*Nanny Grattan and Ashley (age 2)*

well as the computer, had been purchased for my use through a grant at Lakehead University. Therefore I was told that if I decided to pursue other jobs in this field with other companies, the equipment that I had been using would be mine to keep. All I would need to purchase was the computer program Arc/Info. This program at the time ran around ten thousand dollars. I contacted the local ODSP (Ontario disability support program) to see if they would be able to help me out. They were able to help me purchase the rest of what I needed in order to become self-sufficient in my own business. I was then able to open my own business, Anderson Digital Data Inc. One of my bigger clients was the Ministry of Natural Resources (MNR). I was one of many subcontractors working on Ontario Base Maps (OBMs). I continued to run my business, working out of the Lakehead University forestry department and paying a fee to lease my office. My future seemed bright, and I could not have been happier.

Once I got my new business up and running I took a few days off. I was scheduled to go into the hospital to have a few screws removed from the plate in my right upper thigh that had been bothering me. That plate had been in my leg for many years, and the screws had loosened and were close to the skin surface. When I ran my finger down the side of my leg I could feel them. While I was in the hospital I ran into Stan. He was still working at St. Joseph's General Hospital. He happened to be working evenings on that floor in the housekeeping department. When he found out that I was a patient, he came to my room for a chat every night. Rina's sister in-law Donna came to visit me, and Stan had come into my room to talk. When he left, Donna asked, "Who's that? He's cute, with those beautiful blue eyes. There's someone for you."

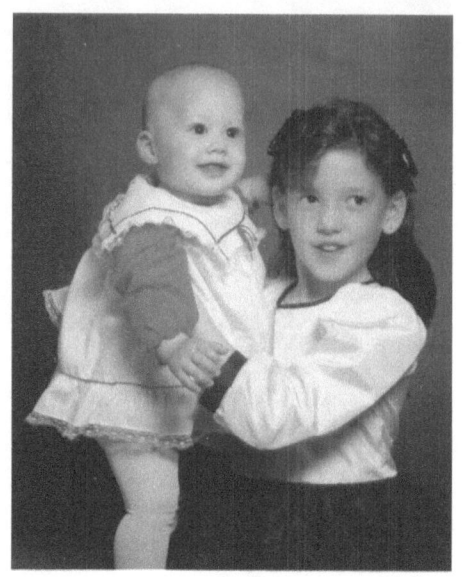

*L. to R. Rachel and Amie*

I said to Donna, "Yes, except he's married with two children. So I think I just have to keep looking."

By then, Stan was divorced and in a new relationship. He told me that he had remarried a few years earlier and that they had just had a little girl.

Mom also went into the hospital that year for a bladder repair. This is a fairly common procedure for women who have had several children. During the surgery the doctor decided to take out her uterus. This had not been discussed prior to surgery, but whatever the reason the doctor felt he should remove it while doing the bladder repair. Mom was fine with this decision because she certainly did not want any more children. Like all organs that are removed, the uterus was sent for a biopsy. The results showed the beginning of a type of uterine cancer that the doctor said would not have been detected until it was too late. Mom and all of us were so thankful that the doctor had made this bold decision. Mom recovered well and was back to her old self before long.

# Chapter 12

## *Moving Out*

I lived with my parents until I was twenty-four. By then, I knew the time had come for me to have a place of my own and decorate things the way I wanted. Living at home was fine, but the time to prove to myself that I could manage on my own had finally arrived. At the time, I was taking my GIS training at Lakehead University. I had become good friends with Ulf, the young professor who had joined the forestry department. He had been looking for an apartment and happened to choose the same building that I had been considering. One of the reasons I was so drawn to the building was the location, which was just down the road from my parents' place. I knew that I would still need a lot of support from them, now more than ever. The neighborhood was familiar, and I was still close enough to my parents in case I needed their assistance. Another plus for me was that the area had lots of trees, green space, and walking trails. This meant that there was a lot of wildlife, such as deer, foxes, chipmunks, squirrels, and wild birds; there were even some beavers living in a nearby pond.

The apartment was beautiful, with two bedrooms, a nice kitchen with a separate dining area, a large living room, a storage room, a deck, and quite a large bathroom. The bathroom was one of the biggest I had ever seen in an apartment. Even with the door shut, there was plenty of room for my wheelchair. Bathrooms always tend to be an issue for me because most of them aren't big enough to accommodate my wheelchair and still allow me to close the door. I called the landlord to ask a few questions about the apartment, and I happened to mention that I used a wheelchair. She immediately told me that the building had no elevator and that there were no available units on the first floor. I was shocked because I knew for a fact that there was an elevator in the building. I was disheartened to know that she was telling me a lie; I think that she'd made up her mind about who should be allowed to live in this particular building. It was even more hurtful because I had gone to high school with her and she had married a minister.

When incidents like this happen, and they continue to happen to me from time to time, I feel sad, not so much for me but for the attitudes and misconceptions that people have. Having to face these attitudes time and time again can become difficult, but overcoming them has made me a stronger person. We all know that saying, "When life gives you lemons, make lemonade." We have to take negative situations and put the best possible spin on them.

The building filled up quickly, being such a nice place with fairly large, modern apartments. Before long, every unit was spoken for, so I went on a waiting list. My friend Ulf from the university was going to let me know when a unit became available, and I decided then that would be my chance to make my move.

I knew that moving out of my parent's home would be a difficult decision for Mom to accept because we were close and spent so much time together. I was not quite sure how to tell her about my plan, so I waited until the last moment. That was a bad idea. This would become the first time in my life that my Mom and I disagreed about anything.

What was even worse was that she found out about my plan from Ulf. He happened to call the house one morning to talk to me about the apartment. I had already left for work, so he had a chat with Mom and told her, really quite innocently, that I would be moving. Ulf said,

"Oh, hi, Mrs. Anderson. I just wanted to tell Heather that a unit has become available at my apartment building for her to move into."

My mother said, "Thank you, Ulf, I will let her know." She hung up the phone feeling a bit confused and shocked because that was the first that she had heard about my plans to move, and I had not told her myself. When I got to work that day Ulf came to me and said, "Heather, I tried to phone you this morning to tell you there is an apartment available for you. So I told your mom to let you know."

I said, "You told my mom?!"

Ulf replied very innocently, "Yeah, we had a chat about the apartment." I remember my heart dropped at that moment, and I said, "Ulf, you idiot. I haven't even told my parents that I'm moving out! Now you just did that for me."

Ulf replied, "Heather, you haven't told your parents yet? What's the matter with you, why would you not have told your parents?"

I replied, "Look, Ulf, this is not your fault. I know I should have taken care of all this before, but I just could not seem to find the right moment to break it to them."

Ulf then said, "I'm sorry I told your mom before you could, but I never thought you would have left it this late to tell them. Did you think that they would be mad at you for moving out?"

I said, "No, not that they would be mad, but I know that they will be disappointed that I'm leaving. Every parent has a hard time letting go of their kids."

Ulf said, "Just go home tonight and tell them the truth. Everything will be fine." He laughed as he walked away, shaking his head.

I was anxious and nervous about going home that night to confront my mom. I was not worried about my dad. I knew that he would be fine with the idea, but I knew in my heart that Mom would take it badly.

That night when I got home, Mom said to me in an angry tone of voice, "What's this about you moving into an apartment?"

I said very nervously, "I want to try living on my own, and the apartment building that Ulf lives in would be great for me."

Mom said, "Why did you not say anything about this before now? I just don't understand why you would do this." Mom was clearly upset.

I said, "Look it's no big deal, I'm not a child."

Mom was storming around the kitchen at this point, and she looked at me and said, "I help you with everything that you need. How are you going to manage?"

I replied, "I have to know that I can survive on my own one day. I don't want to live at home the rest of my life!"

We were both extremely upset at this point, and tempers continued to rise. Dad was sitting in his favorite chair in the living room watching television, trying to stay out of our discussion. My dad never usually said too much; he always let Mom handle things with us kids. He just went with the flow. Finally my dad said, "Stop arguing over something as silly as this."

Mom spoke up. "What do you mean "silly"? How is she going to manage?"

Dad said, "Let her go and try living on her own. Like she said, she has to be able to at some point. We are not going to live forever, you know."

Mom stormed out of the room, unconvinced and very upset. For now the conversation was over. Dad and I looked at each other and shrugged our shoulders. He said, "Don't worry. She'll get over it. Go ahead and do what you want. Give living on your own a try."

Mom and I didn't speak much for the rest of that evening. The tension could have been cut with a knife.

I can't blame Mom for reacting the way she did. I should have dealt with moving out in a better way, but I never meant to let things go until the last moment. I guess that I was just trying to find the best time to tell her.

After a couple of quiet days Mom began to accept my decision. She asked, "When do you get the keys to move in?"

I looked up from what I was doing in surprise and replied, "I already have them."

Mom replied, "Well then, let's go see this place of yours." She looked at me and smiled softly.

I smiled from ear to ear and said, "Do you and Dad want to come and see it now?"

Dad spoke up. "You and your mother can go see it together first, and I will see it later. I'm not feeling up to going tonight." He smiled at me with that look that only a daughter can recognize, the look that seems to say, "Way to go, girl! I told you everything would be fine."

I replied, "Thanks, Dad. We'll tell you all about it when we get back." I knew that since he had fallen off a ladder in his workshop a few weeks ago and hurt his shoulder, he was not feeling well. He'd been climbing a ladder and suddenly fell off. I remember him saying, "What the heck is the matter with me lately! I seem to get off balance and just fall." After the fall, Mom made an appointment with the doctor for Dad to find out what was going on with him. We thought maybe he had high blood pressure.

Mom grabbed her coat, I grabbed my car keys, and we were off to see my new place. I felt a huge sense of relief.

Moving out of my parents' home was an important step, and I was looking forward to experiencing an independent life. I really liked the building, the apartment, and the location, and I felt like this option was perfect for me. The apartment building was new, and some areas of complex were still under construction. The building had been under construction back when I was still in high school, but whatever delayed the contractors from finishing sooner was a mystery to me. The front entrance was nice and flat, with no stairs. Another thing I liked about the building was the small size. There were only four floors and fifty-four apartments, which made a more neighborly feeling.

I still relied on other people to help me quite a bit, so I would need some time to adjust to my new environment and find ways to work things out. My oldest niece Mandy wanted to stay with me at the apartment for the first few months until I got comfortable handling things on my own. Mandy and I always spent a great deal of time together. She was very independent at a young age. She was used to being around me; helping out with whatever was needed was never a problem for her. There are only thirteen years between her and I, so in many ways we kind of grew up together. We had become very close friends, not just niece and aunt. Sheila and John both agreed that Mandy could come and help me out for a while. Like most young people, I found moving from my parents' place to be somewhat of a revelation. Doing laundry, cooking, and cleaning were not high on my list of things to do when I lived at home. The first year on my own Mom often helped me with some of the more difficult chores, like scrubbing floors and vacuuming.

Being on my own meant that I was able to have my nieces and nephew sleep over on the weekends. I really enjoyed having the kids around. Both my sisters raised their children in very relaxed ways. I loved having them with me. Amie was a very bright, beautiful, soft-spoken little girl, and Adam was a shy, sensitive little sweetheart with white hair. Ashley had a wonderful connection with animals. She loved helping with my bird or the cat. I had never seen such a young child be so gentle with animals. I used to say her career one day would be in the animal field. Rachel was pure love. She always hugged and kissed me—a real loving little soul. They all called me Heady, because Heather is a difficult name for children to say. My siblings also called me Heady from time to time.

That summer Carol, Rachel, Ashley, and I went to a local strawberry patch called Gammondale Farm to pick strawberries. Carol kept calling me Heady, and before we knew it, the owner was saying, "Oh, Heady, come over here. There are lots to pick here." We thought it was kind of funny because no one ever called me that except my siblings and my nieces and nephew. We got a kick out of it.

My moving away from home relieved some pressure on my mom. As I think back over the years, I can say with all certainty that my mother has always needed to care for someone other than herself. Some people spend their lives being caretakers. My mother is one of those people. She continued to help me out, but she finally had a bit more time for herself. However, life was still not easy. Dad had been experiencing some difficulty with balance from time to time during the past two years. I remember when Mom and I were sitting at the kitchen table talking and my Dad was making a sandwich. He went to the drawer where the utensils were and pulled it open to get a knife. All of a sudden he lost his balance and fell backward, with the drawer in his hands. We were all shocked and upset. Mom helped him to his feet. He said, "I just seem to get thrown off balance so easily." The look on his face said it all; he seemed disgusted and embarrassed when he left the room. Mom and I looked at each other. Neither of us said anything. Dad was diagnosed with deterioration of the cerebellum later that year. Nanny also needed more assistance with her daily chores. Mom became my elderly grandmother's caregiver now that her brother Kenny no longer lived in town. She took on the responsibility of caring for Dad, too. I used to worry that Mom would become ill herself by caring for so many family members, and I often wondered who would take care of her if she got sick. I used to pray that God would keep her healthy and strong. I believe in angels because of my own life experiences and challenges, and I know that Mom must have some very powerful angels watching over her.

I brought my bird Theodore with me when I moved, but Odie the family dog stayed home with Mom, Dad, and my brother. Once in awhile I would go get Odie and bring him to my place, but he was never very content at the apartment. I realized that his place was back at home with my parents.

The building had a No Pet policy, but a lot of people overlooked it and had small pets. One day when Mandy and I were grocery shopping, we noticed that the pet store in the mall had some kittens for sale. Of course I went to look, and we fell in love with the little grey tabby. We held him for a while then put him back in his cage and went off to finish shopping. I could not stop thinking about that little kitty, so when we were finished with the groceries, I went back to the pet store. For ten dollars I acquired the newest member of my family. He had been at home with me for a couple of weeks before I came up with a good name for him. One day Ulf was over, and he said, "Haven't you named that cat yet?"

I said, "No, I haven't found a name that suits him."

Ulf said, "Why don't you name him Gator, like Gatorade, because he certainly seems to be your pick-me-up." Well, the name choice was made—Gator it would be. I could not have given him a more meaningful name. Theo was a yellow cockatiel that loved to be held, and Gator was a kitty on the go. I was not sure how that combination would work, but before long they became buddies. Gator knew his limits with Theo.

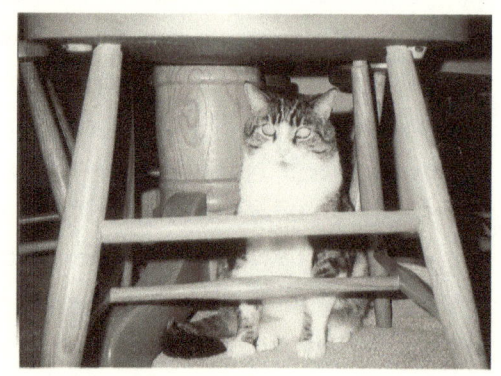

*Gator*

I truly enjoyed living on my own. That summer I wanted to go sailing because I had never been on a sailboat. My dad had a boat when I was young and we would go fishing a lot, but I had never been on a sailboat. I asked Ulf, "Do you want to go sailing with me this summer?"

He said, "Well, I really don't care much for sailboats, but I guess I could." So I booked us for an hour sail. The sun was shining bright that day and the wind had really whipped up, which is of course great for sailing. Ulf and I boarded the sailboat and off we went. I loved the experience of the wind whipping past as we rocked from side to side. I looked over at Ulf and said, "What's wrong with you?" He was looking kind of pale.

He said, "I never told you, but I usually get seasick."

We both laughed and I said, "Do you want to go back to shore?"

He said, "No, I think I'll be fine."

The hour seemed to go by fast for me and I enjoyed every minute, but I don't think Ulf felt the same way.

When winter came Ulf bought a snowmobile, and he wanted me to come and try it out with him. This time I was the not-too-

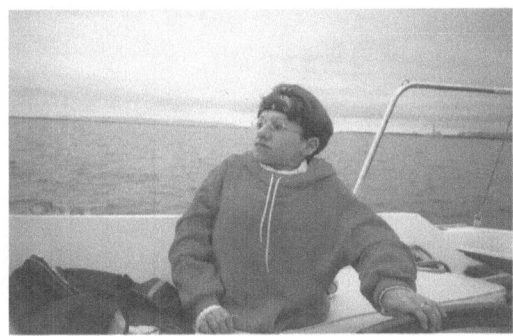

*Heather on sailboat*

keen one. The weather had been so cold that winter, 30 to 40 below. He kept asking me, so I finally said, "Okay, let's go this Sunday." I had fun, but I did freeze, and I think he picked the steepest hills he could find. He must have been getting me back for making him go sailing with me. We had a great time, and I realized I really enjoyed snowmobiling. Ulf had also purchased a motorcycle that spring. He phoned me one night and said, "Heather, how about going for a ride with me on the motorcycle?"

At first I was not sure whether I would have a problem sitting on the motorcycle without falling off. I remember telling him, "Well, as long as the back seat has a bit of a back rest, so that I won't feel like I'm going to fall off." Ulf replied, "Yeah, there is a bit of a back rest. I'll come over, and we can give it a try. If you don't feel safe then we won't go."

It was a beautiful summer evening, with a warm breeze blowing. He helped me on the back, and we both put our helmets on. He said, "Hold on tight to me. If you feel like you're falling, let me know." Ulf got on, started the motorcycle, and off we went. I was having so much fun, with the wind blowing through my hair and the warm sun beating on my face. We must have ridden for over an hour. He yelled to me over the roar of the engine, "Are you all right?"

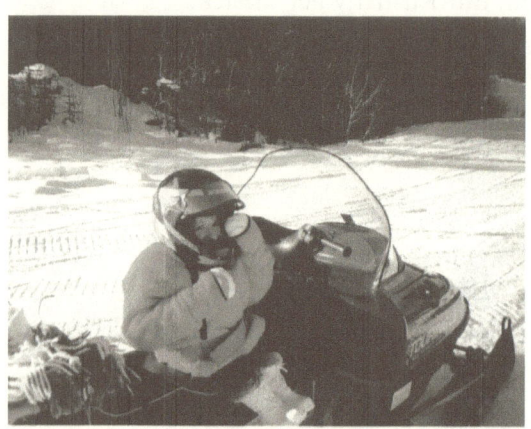
*Heather on snowmobile*

I replied, "I'm fine! This is so cool—keep driving!" What a nice feeling to be able to leave my wheelchair behind and just ride ... Of course we weren't able to stop anywhere because I didn't have my wheelchair, so we just kept riding.

My Uncle Ken and Aunt Pat were in town visiting. They had been coming from British Columbia for a visit every year with their motor home for the past few years. They stayed at Mom's quite often during the month they were in town. Ulf and I stopped by on the motorcycle to show my uncle. He came outside and said, "Look at you! You're riding a motorcycle now! How great is that?" He loved fixing old cars and bikes, so he really took an interest in Ulf's new motorcycle. The two of them must have chatted for an hour about that motorcycle. From that day on, Ulf and I often went for a ride on the warm evenings.

I have had some really interesting and diverse opportunities in my life. During the year after I graduated from high school when I worked at Grandview Lodge Nursing Home, I became friends with Jim Hyder, the fellow who had hired me. About a year after I had been on my own, Jim called to ask whether he could submit my name as a potential interviewee for a television show called *Distant Voices*. The basic premise of the series was that each week someone from the North who had an interesting life or interesting story to share would be interviewed. I was about twenty-five years old at the time and quite unsure why my life would be considered interesting.

Time passed and I forgot all about Jim's request, until one day out of the blue Jim called to tell me that I had been chosen to be interviewed. I was surprised, proud, and afraid because I was going to talk about my life on television. Wow! The time came to do the interview. I was told to meet the crew at the producer's camp, where the episodes were being filmed. This was an exciting experience for me. I realized just how difficult it is to appear on camera. After multiple takes, they finally had enough film for a half-hour episode.

After the tape was edited, the producer sent me a copy so that I could preview it before it was aired. My family, friends, and I had a viewing night. We were all very pleased and proud of the final product; I couldn't believe how good they made me look and sound. A competent and creative editor can do wonders! After the show aired, I felt like a real TV star. Strangers would come up to me in the grocery store and say, "I saw you on television. What a great story!" I was very proud that I had agreed to be interviewed, and I felt blessed that I had the opportunity to share my life story with so many people. That was my first experience of being on TV.

Dad had been slowly going downhill since his diagnosis. He could no longer work. His plan had been for him and Mom to travel a bit when he retired. That was not to be. Gradually he was losing his motor skills. Walking became more difficult, and he was becoming more and more withdrawn. The new truck he had bought two years before now sat in the driveway unused because his eyesight had also been affected, and it was no longer safe for him to drive. Mom had never had a license. She said, "When I was young Kenny started teaching me. I ended up driving his car into the ditch. After that I just could not find the courage to continue learning." When I decided to live on my own, I thought it was important for Mom to learn to drive, so I bought her some driving lessons. She would have been about sixty-four at the time, so she wasn't all that pleased with the idea at first. She thought it over, and because the lessons were a gift, she agreed to give them a try. Beside, the practical side of her didn't want my gift to go to waste. She now says that she can't understand why she never learned to drive sooner, and she doesn't know how she ever managed without her driver's license.

# Chapter 13

## *Hearing Loss*

I'd always known that I might begin to lose my hearing in my early twenties or thirties as a consequence of having OI. In at least three of the types of OI, hearing loss is common due to a calcification of the *stape*, the part of the inner ear that moves and conducts sound. I never gave this possibility much thought as I was growing up because my hearing was fine. That was up until 1990. I was twenty-seven years old when I started to develop hearing problems. At first my ears just seemed plugged, so I would try to clear my ears by pinching my nose and blowing. I thought that if I could just get my ears to pop I would be able to hear well. There was always a crackling sound in my ears when I blew my nose. Finally I was sent to an ear specialist to see whether something could be done.

When it was determined that my problem was due to OI, I was left with two options: wear hearing aids or have surgery to correct the problem. I was not at all keen on wearing hearing aids. I felt like that was one more thing to deal with that made me feel disabled. I wore leg braces for many years while I was doing therapy, and I had always hated wearing those uncomfortable and heavy things. The braces were not practical for me because I knew that I would never have the strength and stability to use the braces and crutches to walk around and do my daily activities, so I preferred using my wheelchair, which made it easier and faster for me to get around. Using my wheelchair also eliminated the greater risk of slipping or tripping and falling, which would inevitably result in one or more fractures.

The idea of wearing a hearing aid for the rest of my life didn't go over well with me. But when I began to have difficulty hearing at work and communicating with others, I finally accepted that I needed to do something. I held off as long as I could, until everyone began telling me how loud my TV was and so on. I also found myself becoming withdrawn and not wanting to go places with other people because I knew that I could not hear half what they were saying. I began to research the surgical procedure that could potentially correct my problem. I found that the procedure was 99 percent successful in restoring normal hearing. Although this condition also occurs in people without OI, the risks of the procedure are greater for a person with OI because the longer the nerves are exposed to the air during surgery, the greater the risk of permanent damage.

I found a doctor in Memphis, Tennessee, who was achieving extremely successful results with laser surgery for patients with OI. The laser minimized the trauma to the auditory nerve. I was eager to have this surgery, hoping to restore my hearing. However, I couldn't afford to have the surgery in Memphis. I obtained the names of several Canadian surgeons who could do the procedure closer to my hometown. I chose a doctor in Ottawa, and Mandy and I flew there for an assessment. Mom was not able to come with me because she needed to stay home to care for Dad. He now needed more assistance than ever with daily routines. Mandy and I spent a great deal of time together, so her coming with me seemed logical. Even though no one in Canada was using a laser to perform the type of ear surgery that I needed, I was assured by the doctor that he could do the surgery. I felt confident and agreed to proceed with the surgery after I was told that there was only a 1 percent failure rate. Well, guess what? I was in that 1 percent! I lost all hearing in my right ear, and because of nerve damage resulting from the surgery, I also was unable to use a hearing aid.

I don't believe that I have ever been more distraught in my life. Everything that I had endured in my life paled in comparison to this distressing situation. I thought that I would never find the strength to pick myself up again—I was devastated. I spent the next three months sleeping on my couch with a candle burning on my coffee table. This seemed to be the only way that I could sleep. I eventually found the strength to look at my situation objectively and consider my next step. A year after the surgery I went to my audiologist, who told me that my only option was to use a hearing aid in my left ear, because the hearing in that ear also was affected. Because there was no nerve damage in that ear, I could use a hearing aid to improve the hearing I had left. I was fitted for one of the smallest digital hearing aids available, which fit right inside the ear canal. Wearing the hearing aid felt awkward at first, but I was delighted that I could now hear well. I had never realized how loud the flushing of a toilet could be!

Once again, things began to turn around for me, and I started to feel more hopeful. Although my hearing has continued to decrease over the years, I try not to think about it. The best that I can do is cross each bridge as I get there. I have to remind myself not to be consumed with worry.

I was asked to do a couple of commercials for the hearing institute that provided my hearing aid. I agreed because I understand how difficult it is for people to accept hearing loss. I was one of them.

# Chapter 14

## *Six Years of Unemployment*

After seven years, the contracts with the Ministry of Natural Resources (MNR) began to decrease because we had finished updating the Ontario Base Maps (OBMs). I began looking for other work in the field, but to no avail. Thus began a six-year struggle without employment. I could have papered the walls of my apartment with all the rejection letters I received. I eventually began applying for any job that came up, even if it was not in my field of expertise. I was becoming more and more aware of just how difficult finding gainful employment was for disabled people.

The year 1991 was a difficult time for a lot of job seekers. My hometown was experiencing many business closures, and many people were competing for very few jobs. Nevertheless, I knew that I had been overlooked for some jobs because of my OI. In one instance, I applied for a GIS digitizing job with a local forestry company. I had done work for them when I was employed at the university. They had praised my work, but when it came time to hire in-house staff, I was not considered for the position because the office was not wheelchair-accessible. I was not told outright that I was not hired because of my disability. Instead, I was told that the company did not want to hire a subcontractor but rather to train their own in-house person. I would have put my plans to subcontract on hold if the full-time job had been offered to me.

Whether I was working in-house or subcontracting for the company would have made no difference to me. In the end I was not offered the position, so I continued to pursue my plans to subcontract by creating my own company. I was hurt when I realized that I had been passed over because of my physical differences despite the laws that state a person qualified to do the job shall not be discriminated against based on disability. The bottom line remains that employers have the right to hire whomever they want for a job, and no one would have revealed that my disability was the reason for my not being considered for the job. In my heart I knew that was the reason.

That year my bird Theo developed a peculiar chirp. After a short time he became unable to chirp at all. I brought him to the vet, who said he seemed fine. He gave me some penicillin to put in his water in case he had an infection. A few nights after our trip to the vet, Theo fell off his perch. I ran to his cage and said, "Theo! What's the matter?" As I reached in his cage and picked him up, he took one big gasp and died. I sat holding him in my hands, stroking his little head. Tears streaming down my face, as Gator looked on. I said, "Gator, Theo is gone." My heart was broken. Judging by how quickly he went, I believe he must have caught a cold, which caused a heart attack. I was deeply saddened. Gator looked for him for a long time. He would go to where Theo's cage was and look around. The two of them had become friends. Ashley also took it hard. She loved coming over to help me out; she would phone and say, "Heady, would you like me to come and sleep over for the night? I can help you do chores. I can clean Theo's cage and help clean up your apartment." I would say, "Yes, Ashley I would love it if you could come and help me." She was great help around the house. I remember her taking Theo out of his cage gently on her finger. Theo would ride around on her head while she cleaned his cage and gave him fresh food. Then we would get in our pajamas, make a snack, and watch a movie. I loved having each of the kids over to spend the night with me.

Through an organization called Therapeutic Horseback Riding, I also started to learn to ride horseback that year. What a wonderful organization. The staff is dedicated to creating an environment that allows disabled people the opportunity to ride. The horses are trained and worked with extensively for this use alone until the handlers are confident that they can trust the horse to stay calm under unusual situations. Every Thursday night I had the opportunity to ride for a

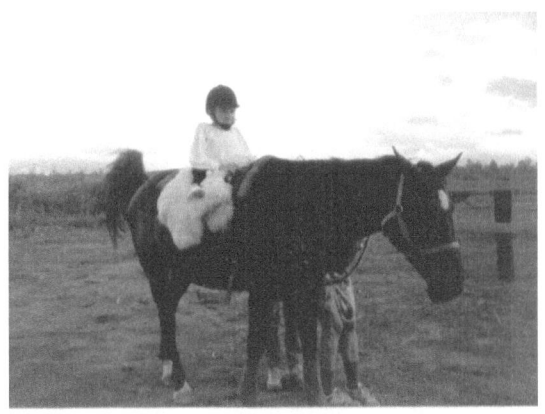

*Heather on Bal*

couple of hours. Horseback riding has become extremely therapeutic for those who are physically challenged. One person led the horse and two stood on each side, making this a very controlled situation. I always felt completely safe, which allowed me to truly enjoy the experience. The time spent on the horse in the outdoors helped me relax and refocus during this difficult time in my life.

Those six years were rough times. I lost everything, and I had to go through a protracted struggle to get back on the Ontario Disability Support Program (ODSP) to pay for my apartment. Because I was living on my own, like everyone else I needed to maintain a job in order to pay the bills and survive. I wasn't going to let my apartment go without a fight. When I had moved from my parent's home several years earlier, I intended to remain independent. I truly enjoyed living on my own; my apartment was my sanctuary, and I felt completely independent. With no job in sight, I was running out of time and funds. If I were going to remain in my apartment, I had no choice but to reapply for ODSP. The decision to go back on ODSP was hard for me to accept. I wanted to remain independent and take care of myself without relying on a disability pension.

Getting reinstated into ODSP was not easy for me. I had been out of the system for so long and acquired so much—my apartment, a car, and household items—that they denied me at first. I ended up waiting almost a year before I could get reinstated on ODSP. One roadblock after another appeared, and each time I spoke with an intake worker I was denied. As the months went by, I tried to survive on what I had saved. My situation left me in dire straits, with no means to support myself. After a year of struggling with this situation I finally spoke to a worker who said, "I can't believe that you have been given this bad rap. I'm sorry; you just happened

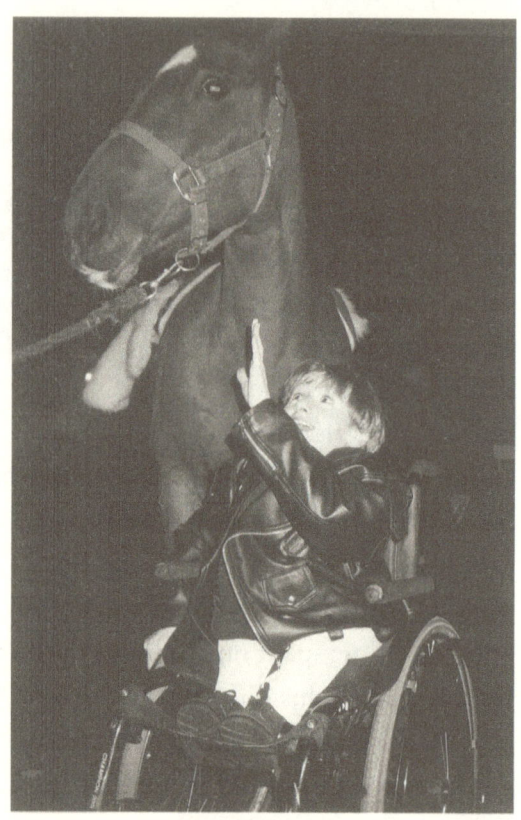

*Heather and Bal*

to be someone that through no fault of your own has fallen through the cracks. The system sometime fails people when they need it the most."

Once I was back in the system, I received $960 per month in assistance, but my rent alone consumed $800 of that. When my contract had ended with the MNR, I had a car loan, car maintenance payments, rent, credit card payments, and expenses for food and utilities. With bills pilling up and no job in sight, I had no choice but to declare bankruptcy. I felt as though my life were over. All the effort that I had put in to overcoming the obstacles in my life now seemed meaningless. I remember thinking that God won't give us more than we can handle, but I truly felt that I had reached my limit. Only my family and friends, who had always believed in me, and Gator, my beautiful little cat, got me through those emotionally rough times.

Two years into my dry spell, Nanny passed away. She had just turned ninety. Even though losing Nanny was hard, I knew that she had lived a full life. She was a happy person who seemed to enjoy life very much, and she loved children. She especially loved having my sisters' children around. Right to the end, she lived life to the max. That Christmas Eve, like every Christmas Eve for the past six years, our family had gone on a sleigh ride, and Nanny still wanted to be part of the fun. The whole family would bundle up in snow suits and blankets. Even the horses were all decked out for Christmas with bells around their necks. We always lucked out with mild weather and big snowflakes that fell softly to the ground. Someone was always pushed off the sleigh and had to run to catch up. Nanny would say, "Heather and I are off limits, so don't push us off." She enjoyed that Christmas tradition so much.

She only spent a few weeks in the hospital at the end. Up until then she had still lived in her own home. A few days before she passed, she and I were talking, and she told me, "You know, Heather, Grandpa came to me last night. He took me by the hand and said, 'I'll be back for you soon.'" She passed a few days later. The last few years she had often told us that she was ready to "go home," as she would say. I remember saying to her one time, "Not yet, Nanny." She replied, "I'll stay as long as I still feel fine. After that I have to go be with Grandpa."

Even though those six years without work and money were difficult, I eventually learned to just let things go. I needed to detach myself from all the material things that we cling to. As long as I had Gator, my friends, and my family, everything was right in my world; in fact, I even began to enjoy whatever life brought my way. I never had a penny in my pocket, I hadn't bought myself anything for ages, and I hardly ever got my hair cut, but I was happy. As long as I had enough food for Gator and me, I simply trusted in a higher power that things would work out, and they always did. I truly learned what it meant to trust in a higher power. I sometimes think back to that time and remind myself of the inner peace that I felt. I am reassured to know that I am not in this alone. Faith is all we really need in this life.

I received a call from Debbie, a friend who had moved to London, Ontario, midway through high school. She called and said, "Heather, I haven't seen you in so long. I'm getting married. Would you like to come to my wedding?"

I said, "I would love to, Debbie. If I can make arrangements to get down there, I will be there." I told my mom that Debbie called, and Mom said, "Why don't you go? I'll give you the money. You could use a bit of fun." I did not want to go by myself so I asked Sheila if Mandy could come with me. She was about fourteen years old and very independent. Sheila said yes. Since Mom was paying for the trip, I wanted to keep the cost down. I asked Mandy, "How do you feel about taking a bus?" Mandy said, "That sounds fun." So off we went. What a disaster! Neither of us had ever taken a bus before. We had always flown or gone by car. We were in for a reality check. The first shock was that the bus was hot, dirty, and crowed. About an hour or two into our journey we discovered that we had the bus driver from hell. He would speed up close to other vehicles on the road and then slam on the brakes, all the while cursing up a storm. Mandy looked at me with big eyes, and I said, "I believe we have a psychotic driver." Everyone on the bus seemed concerned with his behavior, but no one was saying anything. We figured if we said something to him, he might become even more erratic. The next stop was about four hours after we boarded the bus and a new driver took over. Thank God! That part of the nightmare was over. We laugh about this incident every time someone mentions the bus, although it wasn't funny at the time.

We had to change buses at the last stop before our destination. I remember saying to Mandy, "Do you think you will be able to carry me down the bus steps, or should I ask the bus driver to help?"

Mandy answered, "No, don't ask the driver, I can manage." Night had fallen and in the dim light, people were pushing and shoving to make their way down the stairs. We lost our balance and fell. Mandy got up and said, "Are you all right? You didn't get hurt, did you?"

I said, "Mandy, I think I fractured my arm."

She replied, "What! You fractured your arm! What are we going to do?"

I said, "Let's just get into our seat on the bus." She helped me get settled in my seat and put a jacket under my arm to support it. Her face was full of disbelief. She asked, "How bad is it hurting?"

I said, "Not really bad, but I do think that I probably have a small fracture. Don't worry, Mandy. We will be there in a few hours, and Debbie can take us to the ER."

Mandy settled into her seat. The bus doors closed and we were off. I just had to hold on for a few hours. I did not want to upset Mandy too much. She was no stranger to how easily I could fracture, having been around me all her life. For the duration of the bus ride we both sat quietly staring out the window, anxiously awaiting our arrival so our nightmare could end. When we got to our destination and the bus doors opened, there was Debbie, smiling. She took one look at us and said, "What's wrong?

Mandy said, "We think Heather fractured her arm." The smile quickly vanished from Debbie's face, and she sprung into action. She was also no stranger to my fragile bones. She said, "Let's get you right to the ER. Everything will be fine." We got into her car and headed straight for the ER. Her wedding was beautiful, and I sported a lovely white cast that matched the bride's dress. Mandy and I flew home, knowing that we'd never go on another bus trip.

Who would have ever believed that six years could go by without even the slightest prospect of a job? As I entered my sixth year without employment, I decided to do some volunteer work with the Red Cross Plasma Centre that had opened in our area. After a few months, the director asked if I would help at the front desk until the center got past its busy stage. I was pleased that she had asked me and eager to show them what I could do to help. Things went well. Many of the staff and clients suggested that I should apply for a job there. A full-time position with the same responsibilities as my volunteer job came up, so I applied for it. At the same time I ran into a former coworker who had worked in the GIS field with me years earlier. She told me about a GIS opening at one of the large forestry companies in town, Buchanan Forest Products. By this time, I had applied for so many jobs that I figured it would be just another dead end. That said, I still faxed my résumé to the company that evening.

The next day, the director at the plasma centre offered me a part-time job. When I asked her why I had not been considered for the full-time position, she told me that I did not have enough computer experience. That comment was a real slap in the face! If I could run my own computer business doing GIS programs, surely I could handle routine office computer skills. I went home that night feeling quite low, but a message on my answering machine about the GIS job changed my mood considerably.

# Chapter 15

## *New Jobs, New Beginnings*

I phoned my (potentially) new employer back, even though it was ten o'clock in the evening, and he hired me on the spot. I was thrilled.

That was the beginning of a new and positive stage in my life. The job was like a dream come true. I was set up with the latest equipment and Arc/Info software. Better still, they asked if I would be interested in working from home and coming to the office for weekly meetings. This could not have worked out better because I really wanted to work from home. Even though I had enjoyed going into work every day at the Lakehead University, I sometimes found the pace a bit much for me. The idea of being able to pursue my career at home sounded great. They did not care what hours I worked as long as I got the projects completed on time. Everything was looking up: I had a great job back in the GIS field, I could work on my own schedule, and I could be at home with Gator. What more could I ask for?

The pay was good, and for the first time in six years, I felt that my life was renewed. What a nice feeling to finally be able to pay my household bills and get groceries without having to go to my parents or friends for help. I gradually caught up on long-overdue bills and made some changes to my apartment. After six long, grueling years, I was finally back where I had longed to be. Before I knew it I felt like my old self again, and I could see new and wonderful opportunities open up all around me.

Shortly after my new job I got a call from Ulf. He said, "Heather, I have some bad news." His voice seemed serious. "Hans has passed away." I was very shaken, and I yelled, "What do you mean? What happened to him?"

Ulf replied, "Apparently Hans was washing the windows at his home. He had climbed the ladder and suddenly fell to the ground."

I said, "Oh, Ulf! I cannot believe it. I am so shocked."

Ulf said, "Yeah, me too."

The day of the funeral we were all there, Peter, Grant, Ulf, and I. It was a sad time. Hans' death had a profound impact on me. He had played an enormous role in shaping the direction of my career.

After Hans' funeral I went on a short trip to Las Vegas with Rina and John. This fell within the first year of starting my new position. We had a wonderful time together. We went to Vegas because John was going to a convention there for work. So during the daytime when John was at the convention, Rina and I would sightsee. One of our most memorable experiences was when we took a bus from our hotel to the Grand

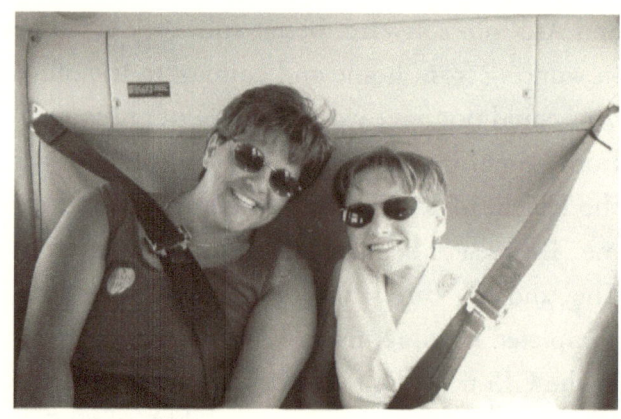

*L. to R. Rina and Heather on plane over the Grand Canyon*

Canyon. When we got there, we then got on a plane that took us over the canyon. What a beautiful experience! Rina and I enjoyed our time together. Because I was not tied into a 9 to 5 job, I was able to enjoy life more.

Working from home and being around Gator all day was wonderful. I enjoyed going out with friends and, as usual, I was still hoping to meet someone to share my life with.

Two years into the new job, another hard blow fell in my life. Dad passed away on October 22, 1998. My father lived with deterioration of the cerebellum for twelve years, but he lost his life to an aneurism. During the past twelve years he became a mere shell of the man he used to be.

Sometimes it's funny how we come to identify other people as the shy one, the strong one, the quiet one, and so on. We kids always

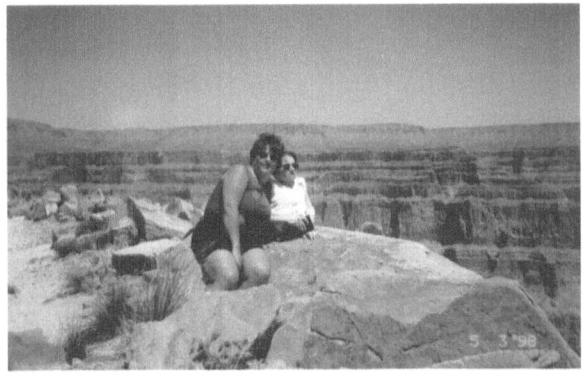

*L. to R. Rina and Heather at the Grand Canyon*

laughed about my sister Carol being the one with the weak stomach. She used to get sick when someone showed her a cut or anything to do with blood, yet when our father passed away I saw a side of her that I had never seen before. When the doctors told us that Dad had about twenty-four hours to live and that there was nothing more they could do for him, everyone thought that I would be the strong one. Despite every-

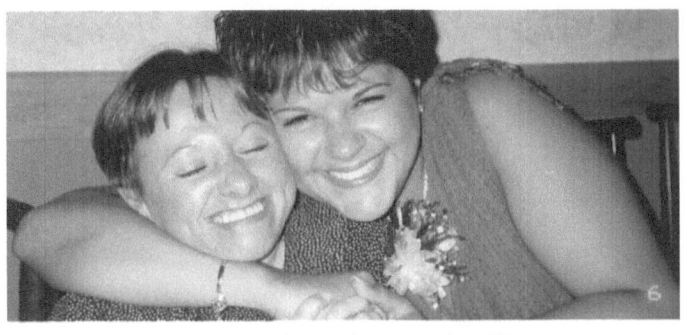

*L. to R. Heather and Rina in Las Vegas*

thing that I've been through in my life, I fell apart and developed a full-blown migraine. Carol became the strong one. She took me to the ER for treatment and listened to me throw up uncontrollably, which we laughed about afterward, because it scared her and the doctor.

Then she'd run back upstairs to be with Dad and the rest of the family. She spent the entire night with Dad while the rest of us went home to catch some sleep. After Carol went home in the morning to freshen up, Mom and Sheila took over and stayed with Dad. He died shortly after she left. She was upset that she hadn't been there when he died, but I know that's how Dad wanted it. She had done her part, and Dad did not want her to be there during his last moments.

No one knows the path that a life will take or how that life will end. Life can be a cruel journey, but I believe that joy, beauty, and meaning can be found in every aspect of life. When I look at the blessings that surround me, I know that I am on this earth for a reason. I will continue to live my life by touching the lives of others.

Losing Dad was hard on all of us. I took a few weeks off work to pull myself together and help Mom with whatever she needed to do. That Christmas we decided that the family would forego our regular sleigh ride on Christmas Eve. We figured changing our routine might ease the pain of our first Christmas without Dad. At times we would find ourselves laughing and joking with each other, and then one of us would recall a funny time with Dad. Instantly we'd be jolted back to the stark reality that he was gone. Never again would we come home to see him sitting in his favorite chair in the living room, bask in his warm smile, or have the opportunity to create new memories. The realization of how short and precious life really is never hit home harder than then, but we realized that our family would always be there for one another until the end.

In the weeks after Dad's funeral, I remember saying, "This is going to be the year I find my mate. After all the sorrow of losing Dad, we all need something to celebrate and feel good about." My sisters would say, "Yeah, sure you will, Heather." I had been saying this for so long that everyone just kind of shrugged it off.

I always knew that one day I'd find that one special person in my life. I can't explain what I wanted in a partner, but I did know that what he did for a living or how successful he was in his chosen career would not be important. All I really knew was that I wanted a special connection with someone who could fill a void in my life.

I was thirty-four when I found the person that I had been hoping for. I had lived on my own for ten years, and even though my life as a single woman was full, I knew that I did not want to spend the rest of my life alone. On January 12, 1998, Mom and I stopped at a local grocery store to pick up a few items for supper. I was feeling quite good about the direction I was headed at that time in my life. I was doing GIS work for a major forestry company; I had made long overdue changes to my apartment; and for the first time in six years, I could buy a few things for myself. Life was finally going my way.

I didn't shop at this particular grocery store very often, but for some unknown reason it's where I chose to go that day. We were looking over the selection at the meat counter when we heard someone say, "Hi, Heather." Mom and I looked up and saw Stan. Stan and I had worked together at the hospital about fifteen years earlier. I had liked him and thought he was very handsome. I knew he liked me too. He used to go out of his way to talk to me, but he was much older than I was. When we worked together that year at the hospital I was nineteen, and he was married and had a son. Perspectives seem so different when we're young and we meet someone who's a few years older. Stan seemed secure in his life and so much more mature than I was. I was really just starting my life and had no real direction.

Over the next fifteen years we would bump into each other every so often. I never thought that Stan and I would date. That seemed so unrealistic.

Back to the grocery store … We chatted for awhile and caught up on the news in each other's lives. I recall asking him, "How are your wife and the kids doing?"

He replied, "Unfortunately, we divorced about two years ago. My daughter is with her mom and my son is with his mom, my first wife. Remember, this was my second marriage."

I said, "I know, you told me back when I was in the hospital that you had remarried. I am sorry to hear that things have not worked out for you."

He said, "I'm living with my parents until I regroup from the divorce. Are you married or seeing anyone?"

I replied, "No, I'm still looking."

Stan then asked, "Would you like to go out for coffee or dinner one evening?"

I replied, "Sure."

Stan said, "What's your phone number?"

I told him my number and we both headed to the checkout. He didn't write it down, so I was positive that he would forget it. I never gave it any more thought until I got home and heard the phone ringing. I rushed to answer. "Hello." I said.

The person on the other end said, "Hi, how are you?"

"Stan!" I said, "Is that you?" To say that I was shocked at how quickly he called me is an understatement.

He replied, "Yes! I really would like to get together with you and catch up on things."

I said, "I would really like that as well."

Stan said, "How about this Friday?"

"This Friday sounds great. Would you like to come to my place?"

Stan answered, "I will bring the wine, and we can order a pizza. What time would you like me to be there?"

I said, "How about 6 PM?"

"Sounds good. I can hardly wait."

I replied, "Me too," and I gave him my address and hung up the phone.

At precisely six o'clock Friday night, Stan was at my door. We had a great time together that evening. We really enjoyed each other's company. When he asked, "Would you like to see me again?" I said, "Yes, I think that would be wonderful."

He smiled with the shyness of a little boy and said, "Goodnight."

We became inseparable after that. I knew that the empty place in my life was gone. Stan was the right person for me. After we got more comfortable with each other, I asked him how he had remembered my phone number that day in the grocery store. He told me that he had asked one of the cashiers to write the number down for him. He called me right away before he lost his nerve. We often talk about the days when we worked together at the hospital. Stan said that he thought I was the cutest girl right from the first day he had seen me drive into the parking lot at the hospital. I told him that I had always been attracted to him too.

I never believed that I would become involved with anyone who had already been married … and had children. I felt that those were not options for me, but once Stan and I got to know each other I realized how narrow-minded I had been. Before long, I knew that if our relationship was meant to be, it didn't matter what had happened in the past. The future … our future … was more important than the past.

Our relationship continued to develop, and all of my dreams seemed to be coming true. We went for long romantic walks and talked until the sun came up. I could see that Stan had a beautiful soul. He had a great respect for nature and all life, right down to his love for animals. Stan and Gator took to each other immediately. Stan's love for my Gator meant a lot to me.

The relationship moved along quickly. About two months into the relationship, I learned that Stan was an alcoholic. At that moment my whole world was shattered. How could this be? How could something that seemed so right have such a terrible reality? Was I dreaming? How could this be true? After the initial shock wore off, I pulled myself together. We talked openly about his problem and what it meant for us and our evolving relationship. I spent the next few weeks talking to everyone who knew him well, including his ex-wives. I needed to know the depth of his addiction so that I could make a rational decision about continuing or abandoning our relationship.

I know that most people would say that addiction is an automatic deal breaker, but I could not just walk away based on what society dictates we should do. I had lived my whole life rising above obstacles and stereotypes, so I wanted to make my decision based on what I felt was right for me. How could I walk away from a relationship that seemed so right? I confronted Stan about his addiction and told him that the only way I would continue this relationship was for him to get help. But did he want help? After endless hours of talking, he assured me that he wanted help to put his addiction in the past and get on with his life.

I took the next few weeks to sort things through and come to a decision that I could live with. I spent many days asking myself why God would allow this crisis in my life. I was angry, and for the first time in my life I was angry with God for having dealt me this hand. Why would he finally bring me this wonderful soul and then destroy our relationship in this way? Stan had everything that I wanted in a partner, but his being an alcoholic was not part of the equation. My family and friends were worried that I was getting myself into a bad situation. Mom liked Stan a lot, but she also knew how serious the situation was. She trusted me enough to know that whatever decision I made would be what was best for me.

Stan asked whether I would support him and wait for him if he went into rehab. I agreed that I would, so we began his journey toward recovery together. Against most people's better judgment, including my own, we set out on the rocky road to his sobriety. I knew that the journey would not be easy, and I was fully aware that I might be setting myself up for heartache, but I had to give it my best effort. Each time he slipped back into his addiction he became someone I did not know and did not want to know. I remember telling Mom that I felt as though I were mourning for him each time he relapsed. The grip of addiction, which is never far from any addict's life, would once again take hold, and the man I fell in love with would be gone for a while. Physically I could see him and hear him, but it was not him. I knew that he was in there … somewhere … and I desperately wanted him back. Through two rehab stays and a few setbacks along the way, it was the best of times and the worst of times.

Stan came into my life when I least expected it, and he filled my heart and soul with a sense of peace and love. He nurtured the part of me that needed it so much, and I believe that we were brought together for a reason. I believe that what we have found in each other has given us the ability to rise beyond any obstacles.

Mom had more surgery the year after Stan and I were together. She had had a cough since the time of my father's death. Mom was never one to get sick very often,

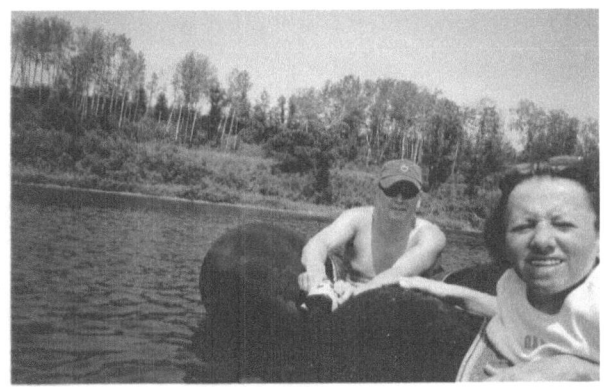

*Stan and Heather tubing*

and she always seemed too busy to worry about herself. Now that Dad was gone she said, "I guess I should go to the doctor and see why I can't seem to get rid of this cough." While she was at the doctor's she mentioned that she had a sore side from time to time. The doctor sent her for an ultrasound and found a mass on her bowel. Surgery was scheduled to remove it. The mass was cancerous. Luckily the mass was contained, and the doctor was able to remove the cancerous part of the bowel and reattach the remaining part, and all was fine. Treatment beyond surgery was not necessary. She would need to have colonoscopies every six months for the first five years. We all breathed a sigh of relief and thanked God that someone was watching over her.

After only two and a half years of my new GIS job at Buchanan Forest Products, the job came to an end. My boss at Buchanan said to me, "Heather, we will be downsizing and letting go of some of our staff. I'm sorry to tell you that you're one of them." I was left feeling as if life were never going to be secure again. I had stood in this spot many times before, and I knew that somehow I would get through this. At least this time around I had Stan to lean on.

Stan and I had been together at this point for about a year and half. I was happy in the relationship area of my life, but I was not too happy about being back in the unemployment line. I knew that the GIS positions in my hometown were going to be few and far between. Since I had worked in the GIS field for over fifteen years, I decided that maybe the time was right for me to switch to something new.

While watching television late one evening, I saw an episode of *Martha Stewart* that caught my interest. She had a fellow on who was doing balloon art. I was very impressed with what he was doing with the balloons. The next day I e-mailed the show and asked how I could find out more about the art of ballooning. This brought me to my next big business venture. I contacted a balloon business called Qualatex, and they sent me all the information I needed on how to get started in the ballooning industry. I told Stan all about what I had discovered and asked him how he felt about us learning this trade and

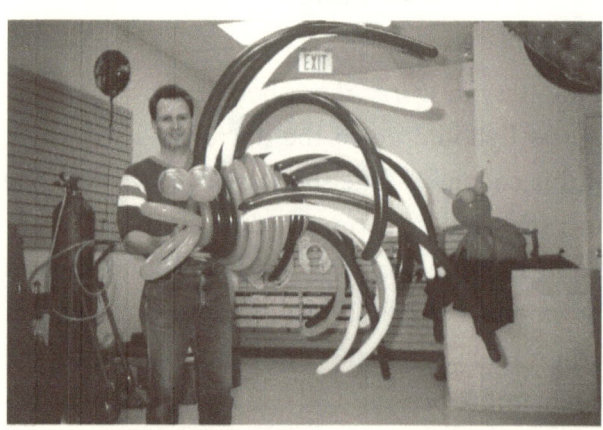
*Stan with balloon sculpture Heather made*

opening a store of our own. He was open to the idea. After he went through rehab, he had taken a job as a tire technician, and this position was not exactly making him happy. Once again I was back in action, and we began to do what was needed to open our shop. We both took to ballooning quite well and really enjoyed learning how to use balloons to decorate. Our hopes were to decorate for corporate events as well as private parties. We had rented a space in a strip mall not too far from my apartment. I took out a small business loan for $10,000 dollars. That was just enough to get us up and running. Since rent was high, we knew that we had to be at least breaking even within the first year or we would not be able to continue. We started off great and even landed a large job with a local mall, decorating for Halloween. Unfortunately, the business did not succeed. We were never able to get completely off the ground the way we had hoped. Rather than put ourselves in the hole, we decided that we would close our shop at the end of our first year when the lease was up.

Determined not to let the financial and emotional efforts go to waste, I decided to do a video on decorating for seasonal events and then promote it on television. I figured that even though we had to close the shop, we could still teach people how to decorate with balloons for their events. I had done the documentary with TVO, and I had also been in two commercials. I was comfortable making a do-it-yourself video on decorating with balloons. I knew a fellow who had been dong his own outdoor life videos for television, so I contacted him and asked if he

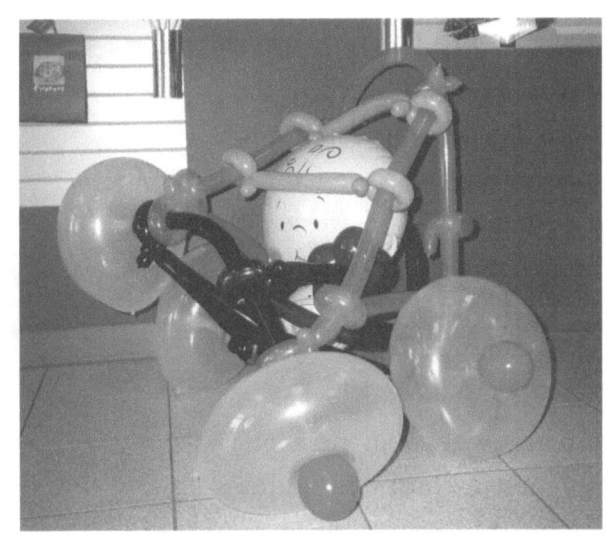

*Balloon sculpture Stan made*

would produce our first video. We could only afford to do the pilot, so after that we began promoting the show. We were able to get our local television station to run it, but we were not having much luck getting a major network interested. My hopes and dreams were big, but this venture soon failed. By this time I was emotionally, physically, and financially drained. I swore that this was the last of my business ventures. I needed the next six months to just sleep and not care about a single thing. Whenever anyone asked me what I was doing now, I would say, "I'm taking early retirement."

My pets have always been my passion in life. When life was more than I could handle my pets were always a source of comfort. I love all animals, domestic or wild. My dream of a perfect world would be to live in harmony with all God's creatures.

Near the end of August 2003, we had to put Odie down. He had reached the ripe old age of seventeen. His hearing had gone about a year before, and we knew he was not able to see much anymore. We had decided as a family that when the day came that he seemed to be in distress, we would then put him down. One evening after dinner he began crying in pain. Mom called me to say, "Odie is crying in pain. We

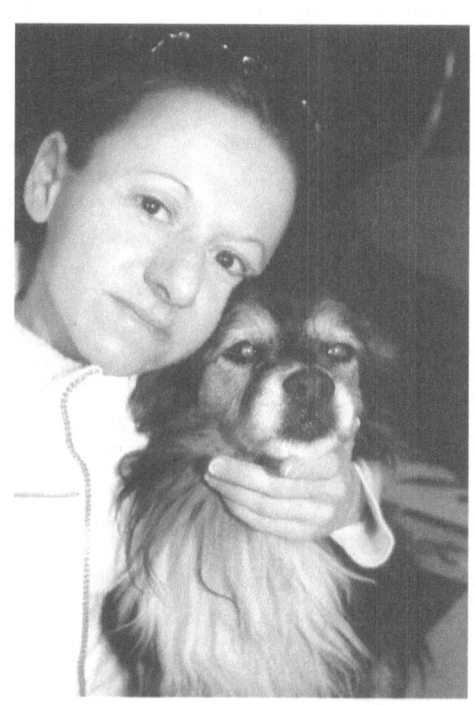

*Heather with Odie,*
*( 6 months before he passed away)*

need to get him to the vet." By the sound in her voice, I knew. It was clear that the time had come to let our beloved Odie go. I got off the phone with tears streaming down my face and said to Stan, "We have to get Odie to the vet. He's suffering. I could hear his howls through the phone. Can you take him? We have to let him go."

Stan rushed out the door to Mom's place. I stayed home, because it was too hard to bear. Our hearts were broken. Odie had been such an important part of the family for seventeen years. Ashley was just a baby when we got him. He had been a wonderful pet. We never had to keep him on a leash because he never left the yard. He would make his circle around the house and then lay by our gate and watch people go by. The entire neighborhood had come to love him over the years. Neighbors asked about him for many months after his passing.

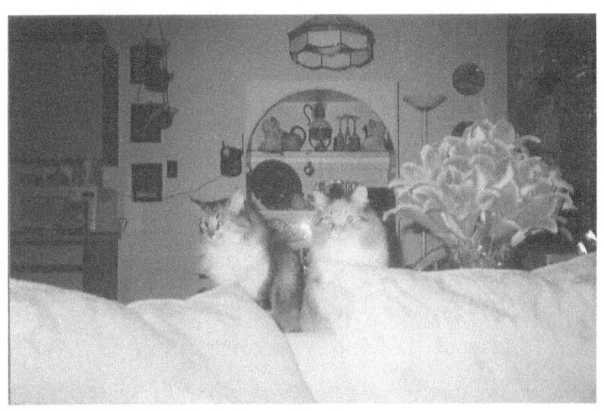

*L. to R. Avery and Allie*

Little did I know that on November 1, 2003, I would lose Gator as well. Everything happened so suddenly, over the course of two days. He was twelve years old when he developed lung cancer. Stan and I were devastated; Gator and Stan had become the best of buddies over the years. His death left a hole in our hearts that I thought would never heal. To work through my pain, I needed to adopt another pet and give my love to another furry baby. Two days later, Stan and I opened our hearts and our home to two little calico sisters. We named them Allie and Avery. Those little bundles of fur helped us to heal one day at a time. No pet ever takes the place of another, but in some small way they do help to ease that pain and show us how to love again. I would like to share one of my favorite poems:

From the book *The Legend of Rainbow Bridge*, by William N. Britton

### The Legend of Rainbow Bridge

Just this side of heaven is a place called Rainbow Bridge.
When a pet dies who has been especially close to a person here on earth,
that pet goes to Rainbow Bridge.
There are beautiful meadows and grassy hills there
for all our special friends so they can run and play together.
There is always plenty of their favorite food to eat,
Plenty of fresh spring water for them to drink,
And every day is filled with sunshine so our little friends are warm and comfortable.
All the pets that had been ill or old are now restored to health and youth.
Those that had been hurt or maimed are now whole and strong again,
Just as we remember them in our dreams of days gone by.
The pets we loved are happy and content except for one small thing.
Each one misses someone very special who was left behind.
They all run and play together, but the day comes
When one of them suddenly stops and looks off into the distant hills.
It is as if they heard a whistle or were given a signal of some kind.
Their eyes are bright and intent. Their body begins to quiver.
All at once they break away from the group, flying like a deer over the grass,
their little legs carrying them faster and faster.
You have been spotted, and when you and your special friend finally meet,
You hug and cling to them in joyous reunion, never to be parted again.
Happy kisses rain upon your face.
Your hands once again caress the beloved head.
You look once more into the trusting eyes of your pet so long gone from your life,
but never gone from your heart.
Then with your beloved pet by your side, you will cross the Rainbow Bridge together.
Your Sacred Circle is now complete again.

(Reprinted with permission of the author. Published 1994. © William N. Britton.
Savannah Publishing c/o LikeMinds Press, Inc.)

I tell everyone that when my time comes to leave this earthly life, they'll find me just on the other side of heaven at the Rainbow Bridge.

# Chapter 16

## *Where I Am Now*

S
tan decided to go back to school in the health care field, and I decided that it was time for me to get serious about writing my book. I was sure that I had more than enough to write about. At the age of forty-five, after a lifetime of challenges, I began to think that perhaps this book would become my one big success. None of my business ideas had ever given me the financial security that I had hoped for, but I would not change a single thing if I had the chance to do everything all over again. Some people spend a lifetime doing things that are safe and never step outside the box. At the end of my life, I don't want to look back and wonder why I hadn't tried all the things that I had wanted to. I know that living my dreams has left me vulnerable at times, but I will never forget the journey nor regret the failures. Life is not about failure or success, wealth or poverty, praise or criticism; it is simply about what we learn about the world, ourselves, and others during our journey, and the gift that we receive is enriched lives. At the age of forty-five, I feel as if I'm the richest person in the world.

I don't see much of the friends that I went to high school with these days. Once in awhile we might run into each other and catch up on things. Ulf got married a few years ago; between his job and personal life, I'd say he's fairly happy. Lori and I don't see too much of each other. I guess we got wrapped up in our own lives. She did get married, and they have one son. She continues to be a busy working mom. We see each other from time to time and try to keep up with each other's lives. She will always be special to me, no matter how often we see each other. Our friendship has survived the test of time, and we share an unspoken certainty that we will always be there for each other, just a phone call away. My friendship with Rina has continued to flourish, and we've shared much laughter and many tears since those high school days. She and John still live in the same house on the next block from my family home. They have two children. Their son is completing his last year in pharmacy, and their daughter has completed college and is working in her field. Some people are destined to cross paths in life just once, but I believe that Rina and I will walk our life paths together. If good friends are golden, Rina is platinum. I thank God that she came into my life and that she is my best friend. She will always hold a special place in my heart.

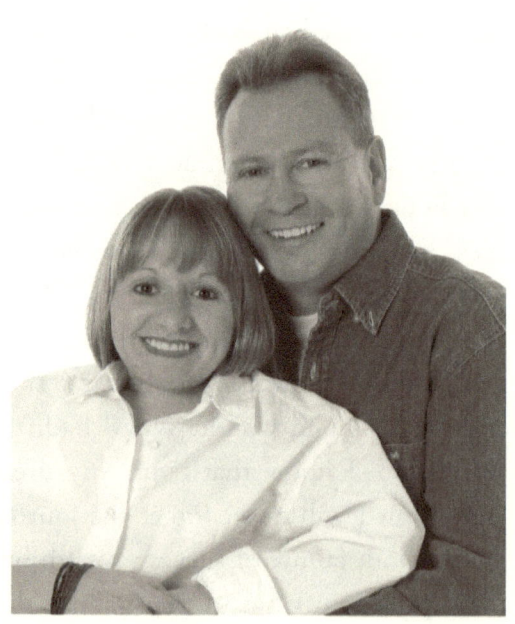

*Heather and Stan, 2009*

Stan and I are now in the tenth year of our relationship. He continues to ground me in a world that can be so harsh. His love for me glows like the brightest light I have ever seen. He is very proud of our relationship, and it shows in everything that he does. I do not nor will I ever regret my journey with Stan. He has taught me the depth of love. We don't look back, nor do we live in the past. Instead, we try to remember the lessons that life has taught us this far, and we strive to be better people.

As I mentioned earlier, I grew up thinking that I would meet my Prince Charming, get married, and have children. Well, I did meet my Prince Charming, but as for marriage and children, the plans changed a bit. As my life progressed and I began to achieve goals that were important to me, I also began to realize that marriage and children weren't as important to me anymore. I just realized that they weren't what I wanted or needed. Many people have commented, "Oh, it's too bad that you can't have children." That's typical stereotyping of people with disabilities. Despite my OI, I could have had children if I had chosen to. OI does not have any bearing on a woman's decision or physical capacity to have children. If we live our lives being true to our own desires, we can find happiness.

Stan and I are very happy, and our life together is fulfilled and fulfilling, despite the fact that we do not have children together and we're not married. Stan's two children from his past marriages are a joy in my life. His son is now twenty-eight years old and has completed a degree in nursing. Work keeps him busy, as does his first home, which he purchased last year. Stan's daughter is eighteen years old and graduated June 2009 from high school. She will be starting her first year of college this fall. I enjoy having his children in my life, and both Stan and I look forward to the future. Perhaps we may choose to marry someday, but for now, I like our life just fine. Stan and I love each other, and to us, that's all that really matters. As for children—I don't feel that I missed out on being a parent. The time I spent with my nieces and nephew as they were growing up allowed me to share in the experience. They are all grown up now and starting families of their own. Mandy turned thirty-two this May. She remains the same strong and independent soul she always was. She and her partner are expecting their first child. They live just outside of Toronto, where she is currently working full-time as a nurse. When she came home for a visit recently, we all eagerly gathered around the television to watch the ultrasound video of her baby boy. You'll never believe when he's due: September 26, 2009. My birthday!

Adam and Amie will be both turning twenty-nine. Adam is engaged to be married and works at Bombardier Plant making streetcars, where his dad also works. His shy, gentle, and loving personality remains to this day. Amie went to university and is living and working in the Toronto area. Her stunning beauty and soft-spoken manor are more prevalent today than ever before. Ashley will turn twenty-three this year. Those big, bouncy curls that were once her crowning glory are long gone, but her beautiful, gentle, caring soul comes through more each day. She is currently working as an animal groomer. I know without a doubt that she is fulfilling her calling to work with animals. She could not be happier. Rachel will turn twenty-one this fall. She will be returning to Lakehead University in September to finish her studies. This summer she will return for a second time to a third world country to help where help is needed. She is our genuine little humanitarian. I truly enjoyed watching my sisters' children grow up and I feel lucky to have been able to share that experience from the time they were born. I was fortunate to have been able to create such special bonds with them when they were children. I will cherish the memories of those days for the rest of my life.

As for my siblings … well, what can I say? They continue to grow older each day along with me, but I still get to say that I'm younger. Our journey together has been incredible. We have and will continue to share in each other's lives in both the worst of times and the best of times. I would not want it any other way. As we all have come to know, life is a challenge at times for all of us, but I've always loved a challenge. I still like to say that I'm three feet tall, but actually I'm only two foot ten inches We'll just round that off to an even three feet.

On March 17, 2006, we celebrated Mom's eightieth birthday with a surprise party attended by more than eighty friends and family members. This was a wonderful celebration of a life that continues to be full and rewarding. She gave up driving when she turned eighty-two. Mom still lives in the family home we all grew up in, and Mr.

and Mrs. Paavola still live across the street. Each time I go home I find myself lost in the wonderful childhood memories that now seem so long ago. This year Mom turned eighty-three, and she continues to be an inspiration to all.

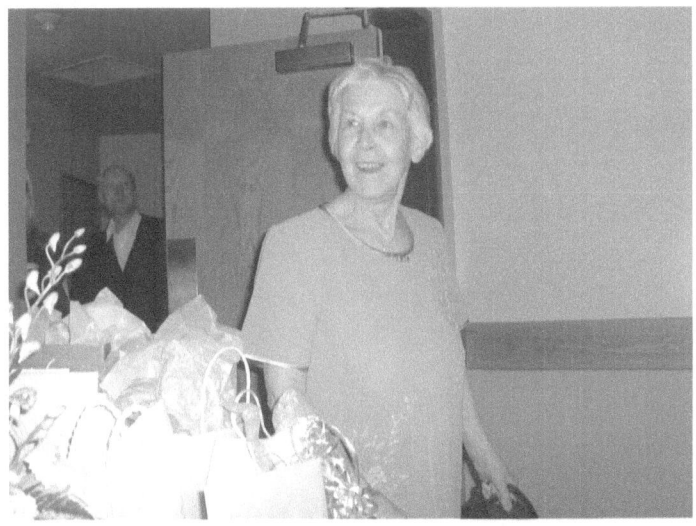

*Mom entering her 80th surprise party, 2006*

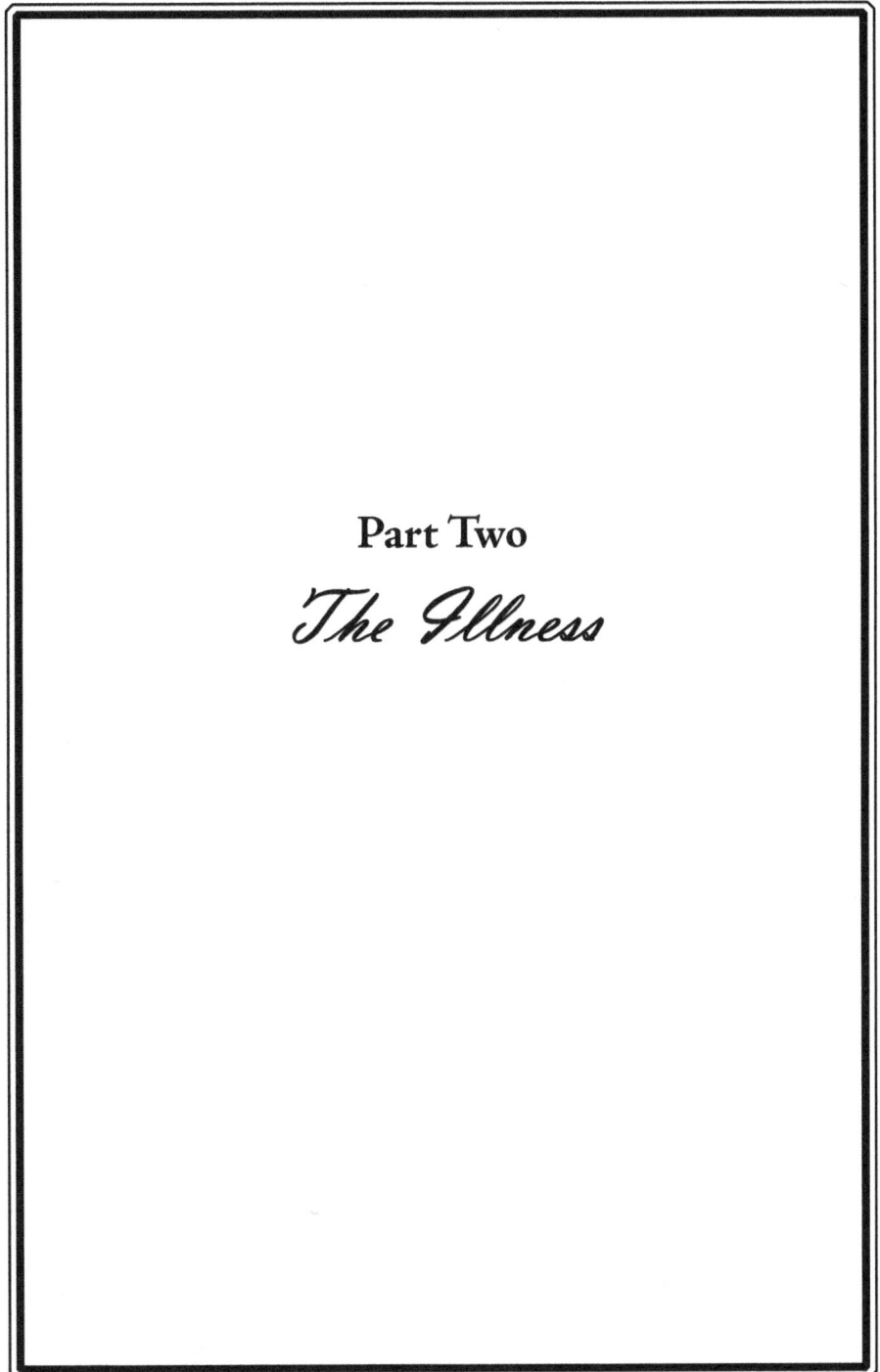

# Part Two

*The Illness*

# Chapter 17

## *What is OI?*

*(Information provided courtesy of the Osteogenesis Imperfecta Foundation.)*

Osteogenesis imperfecta, or OI, is a condition that few seem to know about, yet every day, between one and three children are born with OI. I believe the time has come to bring OI to the forefront, creating necessary public awareness to raise much-needed research money to help battle this debilitating condition.

### Definition

Osteogenesis imperfecta (OI) is a genetic disorder characterized by bones that break easily, often from little or no apparent cause. A classification system of different types of OI is commonly used to help describe how severely a person with OI is affected. For example, a person may have just a few or as many as several hundred fractures in a lifetime.

### Prevalence

While the exact number of people affected with OI in the United States is unknown, the best estimate suggests a minimum of 20,000 and possibly as many as 50,000.

### Diagnosis

OI is a result of genetic defects that affect the body's ability to make strong bones. In dominant (classical) OI, a person has too little or poor quality type I collagen due to a mutation in one of the type I collagen genes. Collagen, the major protein of the body's connective tissue, is part of the framework that bones are formed around. In recessive OI, mutations in other genes interfere with collagen production. The result in all cases is fragile bones that break easily. It is often, though not always, possible to diagnose OI based solely on clinical features. Clinical geneticists can also perform biochemical (collagen) or molecular (DNA) tests that can help confirm a diagnosis of OI in some situations. These tests generally require several weeks before results are known. Both the collagen biopsy test and DNA test are thought to detect nearly 90 percent of all type I collagen mutations.

A positive type I collagen study confirms the diagnosis of dominant OI, but a negative result could mean that an existing collagen type I mutation was not detected; or the patient has a form of the disorder that is not associated with type I collagen mutations; or the patient has a recessive form of OI. Therefore, a negative type I collagen study does not rule out OI. When a type I collagen mutation is not found, other DNA tests that check for recessive forms are available.

## Clinical Features

The characteristic features of OI vary greatly from person to person, even among people with the same type of OI and even within the same family. Not all characteristics are evident in each case. The majority of cases of OI (possibly 85 to 90 percent) result from a dominant mutation in a gene coding for type I collagen (types I, II, III, and IV in the following list). Types VII and VIII are newly identified forms that are inherited in a recessive manner. The genes causing these two types have been identified. Types V and VI do not have a type I collagen mutation, but the genes causing them have not yet been identified. The general characteristics of each known type of OI follow:

## Type I

- Most common and mildest type of OI
- Bones fracture easily. Most fractures occur before puberty
- Normal or near-normal stature
- Loose joints and muscle weakness
- Sclera (whites of the eyes) usually have a blue, purple, or gray tint
- Triangular face
- Tendency toward spinal curvature
- Bone deformity absent or minimal
- Brittle teeth possible
- Hearing loss possible, often beginning in early twenties or thirties
- Collagen structure is normal, but the amount is sub normal.

## Type II

- Most severe form
- Frequently lethal at or shortly after birth, often due to respiratory problems
- Numerous fractures and severe bone deformity
- Small stature with underdeveloped lungs
- Tinted sclera
- Collagen improperly formed

## Type III

- Bones fracture easily. Fractures often present at birth, and X-rays may reveal healed fractures that occurred before birth.
- Short stature
- Sclera has a blue, purple, or gray tint
- Loose joints and poor muscle development in arms and legs
- Barrel-shaped rib cage
- Triangular face
- Spinal curvature
- Respiratory problems possible
- Bone deformity, often severe

- Brittle teeth possible
- Hearing loss possible
- Collagen improperly formed

## Type IV

- Between Type I and Type III in severity
- Bones fracture easily. Most fractures occur before puberty.
- Shorter than average stature
- Sclera are white or near-white (i.e., normal color)
- Mild to moderate bone deformity
- Tendency toward spinal curvature
- Barrel-shaped rib cage
- Triangular face
- Brittle teeth possible
- Hearing loss possible
- Collagen improperly formed

Studying the appearance of OI bone under the microscope, investigators noticed that some people who are clinically within the Type IV group had a distinct bone pattern. When they reviewed the full medical history of these people, they found that groups had other features in common. They named these groups Type V and Type VI. The mutations causing these forms of OI have not been identified, but people in these two groups do not have mutations in the type I collagen genes.

## Type V

- Clinically similar to Type IV in appearance and OI symptoms
- A dense band evident on X-rays adjacent to the growth plate of the long bones
- Unusually large calluses (hypertrophic calluses) at the sites of fractures or surgical procedures. (A callus is an area of new bone that is laid down at the fracture site as part of the healing process.)

- Calcification of the membrane between the radius and ulna (the bones of the forearm) leads to restriction of forearm rotation
- White sclera
- Normal teeth
- Bone has a "mesh-like" appearance when viewed under the microscope.
- Dominant inheritance pattern

**Type VI**
- Clinically similar to Type IV in appearance and OI symptoms
- The alkaline phosphatase (an enzyme linked to bone formation) activity level is slightly elevated in OI Type VI, as determined by a blood test.
- Bone has a distinctive "fish-scale" appearance when viewed under the microscope.
- Diagnosed by bone biopsy
- Whether this form is inherited in a dominant or recessive manner is unknown, but researchers believe the mode of inheritance is most likely recessive.
- Eight people with this type of OI have been identified.

**Recessive Forms of OI**
After years of research, two forms of OI that are inherited in a recessive manner were discovered in 2006. Both types are caused by genes that affect collagen formation. These forms include people who have severe or moderately severe OI but do not have a primary collagen mutation.

**Type VII**
- The first described cases resemble Type IV in many aspects of appearance and symptoms.
- In other instances, the appearance and symptoms are similar to Type II (lethal OI), except infants had white sclera, a small head, and a round face.

- Short stature
- Short humerus (arm bone) and short femur (upper leg bone)
- Coxa vera is common (an acutely angled femur head affects the hip socket).
- Results from recessive inheritance of mutation to the CRTAP (cartilage-associated protein) gene. Partial function of CRTAP leads to moderate symptoms, while total absence of CRTAP was lethal in all identified cases.

## Type VIII

- Resembles lethal Type II or Type III OI in appearance and symptoms, except that infants have white sclera.
- Severe growth deficiency
- Extreme skeletal under-mineralization
- Caused by a deficiency of P3H1 (Prolyl 3-hydroxylase 1) due to a mutation to the LEPRE1 gene.

## Inheritance Factors

Most cases of OI (85 to 90 percent) are caused by a dominant genetic defect. This means that only one copy of the mutation-carrying gene is necessary for the child to have OI. Children who have the dominant form of OI have either inherited it from a parent or, when the parent does not have OI, as a result of a spontaneous mutation.

Approximately 10 to 15 percent of cases of OI result from of a recessive mutation. In this situation, the parents do not have OI, but both carry the mutation in their genes. To inherit recessive OI, the child must receive a copy of the mutation from both parents.

When a child has recessive OI, there is a 25 percent chance per pregnancy that the parents will have another child with OI. Siblings of a person with a recessive form of OI have a 50 percent chance of being a carrier of the recessive gene. DNA testing is available to help parents and siblings determine whether they are carriers of this type of gene mutation. A person with a form of OI caused by a dominant mutation has a 50 percent chance of passing on the disorder to each of his or her children. If one parent has OI because of a recessive mutation, 100 percent of their children will be carriers of the recessive OI mutation. Whether any of these children will have OI will depend on their inheritance from the other parent. Genetic counselors can help people with OI and their family members further understand OI genetics and the possibility of recurrence and assist in prenatal diagnosis for those who wish to exercise that option. For more information on OI inheritance, see the OI Foundation fact sheet titled "Genetics," at www.oif.org.

# Chapter 18

## Treatment

There is not yet a cure of OI. Treatment is directed toward preventing or controlling the symptoms, maximizing independent mobility, and developing optimal bone mass and muscle strength. Care of fractures, extensive surgical and dental procedures, and physical therapy are often recommended for people with OI. Use of wheelchairs, braces, and other mobility aids is common, particularly (although not exclusively) among people with more severe types of OI.

People with OI are encouraged to exercise as much as possible to promote muscle and bone strength, which can help prevent fractures. Swimming and water therapy are common exercise choices for people with OI, as water allows independent movement with little risk of fracture. For those who are able, walking (with or without mobility aids) is excellent exercise. People with OI should consult their physician and/or physical therapist to discuss appropriate and safe exercise.

Children and adults with OI will also benefit from maintaining a healthy weight; eating a nutritious diet; and avoiding activities such as smoking, excessive alcohol and caffeine consumption, and taking steroid medications, all of which may deplete bone and make bones more fragile. For more information on nutrition, see the OI Foundation fact sheet titled "Nutrition," at www.oif.org.

A surgical procedure called *rodding* is frequently considered for people with OI. This treatment involves inserting metal rods through the length of the long bones to strengthen them and prevent and/or correct deformities. For more information, see the OI Foundation fact sheet on "Rodding Surgery," at www.oif.org.

Several medications and other treatments are being explored for their potential use in treating OI. These include growth hormone treatment, treatment with intravenous and oral drugs called bisphosphonates, an injected drug called teriparatide (for adults only), and gene therapies. It is not clear whether people with recessive OI will respond in the same manner as people with dominant OI to these treatments. The OI Foundation provides current information on research studies, as well as information about participating in clinical trials.

**Osteoporosis**

Almost all people with OI are *osteoporotic*, because most people with OI do not develop normal bone mass at any age. Women and men with OI can experience additional bone loss, such as age-related bone loss, superimposed on a background of OI. Symptoms of additional bone loss, including osteoporosis, may appear at a younger age than commonly seen in people who do not have OI. This bone loss may lead to a return to the fracture cycles experienced as children.

**Prognosis**

The prognosis for a person with OI varies greatly depending on the number and severity of symptoms. Respiratory failure is the most frequent cause of death for people with OI, followed by accidental trauma. Despite numerous fractures, restricted physical activity, and short stature, most adults and children with OI lead productive and successful lives. They attend school, develop friendships and other relationships, have careers, raise families, participate in sports and other recreational activities, and are active members of their communities.

## Purpose of Rodding Surgery

A curved or bowed long bone is not in itself a reason for rodding unless it gets worse, repeatedly breaks, becomes painful, or interferes with function. Rodding does not always prevent fractures, but the rod will provide an internal splint that can reduce the risk of displacement of the bone. Rodding may allow the person to be more active after a break and avoid prolonged periods of casting and inactivity. This, in turn, can help break cycles of inactivity that lead to fractures. Fractures may also occur in an area of the bone that grows beyond the end of the rod.

For people with OI, rods are preferred over plates and screws to repair fractures. Plates and screws create a very stiff, short segment within the bone. The bone is likely to break above or below the plate, and long-term use can lead to thinning of the bone underneath the plate.

Walking may be improved after rodding surgery in the child who is ready to walk but is held back because of repeated fractures. However, depending on the severity of OI, walking may not be an appropriate goal for every child. Rodding surgery by itself will not guarantee that a child with a severe form of OI will learn to walk.

## Timing of Surgery

The timing of surgery and the type of rods to use will be affected by the size of the bone to be rodded. The bone must have a large enough diameter to accept a rod. Bones in OI may be thin and flat, so they often appear wider in diameter on X-ray than they actually are. Rodding the long bones in the legs is considered when a child with bowed legs pulls up to stand. Age is not an important factor in determining the need for rodding surgery.

Rodding is usually undertaken as a scheduled elective procedure. However, it can also be undertaken soon after a fracture to avoid a second period in a cast. The fracture may provide an opportunity to perform rodding without opening the fracture site.

As the child grows, the decision about when to revise a rod in a bone that is not fractured is complicated and depends on the child's symptoms (whether the rod is painful or protruding) or the likelihood of the bone breaking in the unprotected segment.

## Types of Rods

The small diameter and length of their bones and prospects for bone growth are two important considerations for selecting rods for children with OI. The orthopedic surgeon matches the rod properties to the specific needs of the child or adult, considering bone size and demands placed upon the bone. The rod should be small enough to fit into the bone canal and stiff enough to support the bone. The rod should not be so large or stiff that it completely shields the bone from stress. Some stress on the bone is necessary for developing and maintaining bone density. Telescoping rods are chosen when there is growth potential. They are not indicated in adolescents or in children with "popcorn" physes, or growth plates, because they have little growth potential. Rods can be made of stainless steel or titanium. There are two major types of rods: non-telescopic and telescopic. Surgeons agree that no single rod is appropriate for all situations.

*Non-telescopic* rods do not expand. They are very versatile and are made in many sizes. For children with very short, thin bones, they may be the only option. They are inserted to support the full length of the long bone. Since this type of rod does not grow with the child, it may need to be replaced as the bone grows if bowing occurs beyond the point where the rod ends.

*Telescopic* rods consist of a thinner rod inserted into a larger hollow rod. They lengthen as the bone grows, which may prevent or postpone the need for replacement. However, they are thicker than non-expanding rods and are, therefore, only appropriate for larger bones. The bone must also be strong enough to allow the rod to be "anchored" at either end. This type of rodding surgery often requires incisions around the joints.

The Fassier-Duval rod system approved by the U.S. Food and Drug Administration (FDA) in 2005 is the newest telescopic rod on the market. Developed by an orthopedist with extensive experience caring for children with OI, it is designed to allow for a less invasive surgery and, therefore, a quicker recovery than other telescopic rods.

## Surgery and Bisphosphonates
Research indicates that children receiving bisphosphonates should discontinue treatment before rodding surgery. Treatment can be resumed when healing is well established.

## Surgery and Aftercare
Rodding procedures are most often undertaken in the thigh bone (femur) and shin bone (tibia). Occasionally, the arm bone (humerus) requires rodding as well. The spine may be rodded to reduce a scoliosis. With modern anesthesia, children can undergo surgery for longer periods of time, thereby enabling several bones to be rodded at one time (e.g., the femur and tibia of one leg). Prior to surgery, key topics to discuss with your surgeon include:

- Physical activity prior to surgery
- The length of the operation
- Time in the hospital
- The length of recovery time at home
- The rehabilitation plan

The question of whether or not to limit the physical activity of young children prior to their first rodding surgery frequently comes up. Experience shows that fractures cannot be prevented by being extra protective. It is also very difficult to stop a young child who wants to crawl, pull to stand, or get into or out of sitting on their own. Exercise enhances bone formation and motor development of the child. The child can be allowed to continue his or her usual physical activities, including swimming, prior to surgery, but parents and caregivers are advised that they should not passively place a child who has severe bowing of the leg bones in a standing position.

When rodding surgery is scheduled, the family and surgeon should develop a plan for what to do if the bone breaks prior to surgery. Often the rodding can be done at the time of the fracture.

*Osteotomy* is a surgical procedure that is often part of rodding. It is used to correct curves or bowing of the long bones. It involves cutting and removing thin wedges of bone so that the bone can be straightened.

The length of recovery period is determined by the extent of the surgery, the type of rod, and the patient's age and activity level. Painful muscle spasms are common after surgery and during recovery. Your doctor or physical therapist can suggest techniques for reducing their pain and frequency. For more information about preparing for surgery and caring for a child in a cast, splint or spica cast, see the OI Foundation fact sheet "Preparing for Your Child's Surgery: What Parents Need to Know Before, During and After Their Child is in the Hospital," at www.oif.org.

## Potential Complications

Rodding is major surgery, and as with any major surgical procedure, there are potential complications. Complications from surgery include risks related to general anesthesia and the possibility of fractures during surgery from inserting an IV or positioning the child. Other issues related specifically to rodding surgery include bleeding, infection, rod migration, and mechanical failure of the rod. More serious complications are rare but all should be discussed with the surgeon beforehand. An experienced surgeon can be a key factor toward minimizing complications in the care of children with OI. Even in the absence of complications, rods may need to be changed as a child grows.

## Rod Replacement

A rod that is not causing pain or interfering with function can be left in place for many years. The question of replacing a rod comes up:

- When the rod migrates (moves) into the joint or outward
- When the rod becomes damaged or fails to elongate
- When the child grows
- When new bone deformity occurs

Whether the rod needs to be removed, replaced, or trimmed depends on the quality of the bone seen on X-ray, as well as the presence of pain, or the appearance that a fracture is likely to occur. When a telescopic rod reaches its maximal length and the bones remain straight, the rod may or may not need to be replaced. Two options are available.

- Wait until the bone breaks, and replace the rod on an emergency basis. This will be painful for the patient and stressful for the family.
- Change the rod on an elective basis based on surgical need as indicated by the X-ray. This option requires thorough discussion between the family, patient, and surgeon.

Adults often have rods that were placed during their teen years. It is not harmful to leave an old rod in the bone. It is still an important part of the support for that bone. Rods occasionally become painful in adults. If pain or significant deformity interferes with the person's ability to function, the rod should be trimmed or removed. Removal can be difficult. As part of preparing for this kind of surgery, the surgeon will want to study old records from the original insertion of the rod and prior X-rays whenever possible. The bone probably still needs support, so in most cases, a new rod will need to be placed. Sometimes the bone quality is good enough that a rod can be removed from an adult without replacement. If the adult is no longer walking, rod removal without replacement may be appropriate.

**Fracture Management for Adults**

- The majority of fractures seen in people who have OI are non-displaced and can be managed with immobilization.
- Displaced fractures can be managed with manipulation under general anesthetic followed by immobilization.
- Care must be taken when manipulating OI bone because of the risk of causing additional fractures.
- OI bone is fragile and can easily fracture proximal to a cast of "normal" weight; therefore, fracture immobilization should be with the lightest materials and techniques possible.
- Adults may have intramedullary rods of different ages and types in different long bones. Their placement and condition should be evaluated if a fracture occurs in a rodded bone.
- Use of plates and screws to repair a fracture is rarely recommended for either children or adults who have OI because:

  1. Poor bone quality leads to screw and plate instability.
  2. Plate rigidity can cause bone loss underneath the plate and fractures above and/or below the plate.
  3. Screw holes may add to bone fragility and predispose to new fracture.

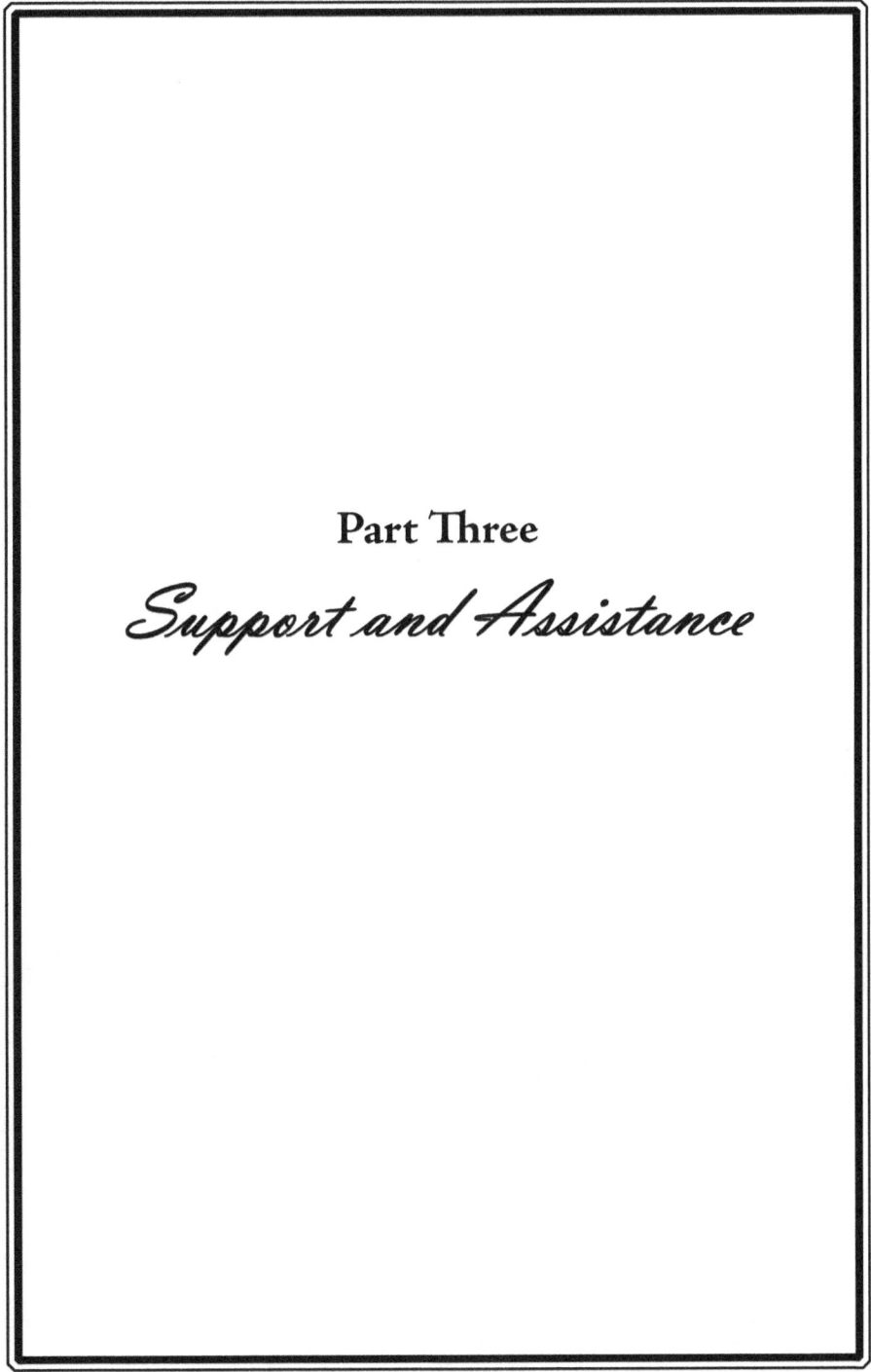

# Part Three

## Support and Assistance

# Chapter 19

## My Goals and the System

I would like to dedicate a big part of the rest of my life to the two worthwhile causes that are most important to me: raising money to help homeless and unwanted animals live a positive, loving existence and raising funds for OI research and awareness. My goal is to start a fund in memory of Gator that can help the loving and loyal pets who cannot help themselves. And through my personal story, I wish to help The OI Foundation, which is the only voluntary national health organization dedicated to helping people cope with OI. Its mission is to improve the quality of life for people affected by OI through research to find treatment and a cure and to provide education, awareness, and mutual support. The OI Foundation was established in 1970 by a small group of parents who met in Chicago to discuss OI. They banded together to stimulate public and professional interest, support families, and encourage research. Today, many of the people who serve on the board of directors and oversee the OI Foundation's operation have OI themselves or are the parents of children with OI.

### Research

Since 1970, the OI Foundation has doubled the funding for research every five years, for a total investment of more than $2 million. Funding for postdoctoral fellowships is available to encourage new investigators to begin a career in OI research and to seed grants for preliminary research. All applications are reviewed by the OI Foundation's Scientific Review Committee, which includes many distinguished OI researchers and clinicians. The potential for results in OI research is growing, with recent advances in gene therapy, a new diagnostic test, and drug therapies under study.

## Education

The OI Foundation's principal educational event is the biannual national conference, which provides close to five hundred people with medical, research, and coping information. For many, it's the first opportunity to meet others who are living with OI. In addition, the foundation is continually developing new information resources in response to the needs of families, individuals, and professionals working with those affected by OI. Topics include schooling, pain management, psychosocial needs of the family, child abuse, fracture management, and osteoporosis.

## Awareness

The OI Foundation strives to build public awareness and generate additional support among individuals, community organizations, public agencies, and medical professionals. Up-to-date information on OI, ranging from medical issues to daily living strategies, available via phone, Internet, fax, and mail, is available. The foundation also reaches out with print publications, press releases, videos, and the Web site.

## Mutual Support

Improving the quality of life is a continuing challenge that the small group of staff and enormous army of volunteers work constantly to achieve. From hosting support groups in twenty-one states and expanding resources, to hosting an online chat room or raising funds, OI Foundation volunteers provide quality support services to people with OI. When people stand together and are committed to a cause, they can make amazing things happen.

I would like to address some of the issues that people with disabilities are faced with when they have no other choice but to live on a fixed government-assistance income. I strongly feel that it is time that these issues be brought forward and that all levels of government take action. I was fortunate that my disability did not hold me back and that I had a supportive family that encouraged me to continue my education. I was able to build a career and maintain my independence, but even so, I was often caught in this vicious trap. I've experienced the obstacles firsthand, and that is why I want to speak out. Life is uncertain; in the blink of an eye, anyone can become disabled and find themselves in the predicament of a physical or mental challenge. Remember, one does not have to be born with a disability; it can happen to anyone at any time.

First and foremost, there needs to be a major change in the basic structure of the Ontario Disability Support Program (ODSP). For those of you who are unaware of ODSP, let me explain. Persons with disabilities who are eighteen years of age and older may be eligible for income support under the ODSP Act, regardless of whether they were disabled from birth or later in life. When I turned eighteen, I started receiving a small stipend. I was still living at home and going to school. Once I got my first job, I was taken off the system. There was a time when earnings were subtracted dollar for dollar from ODSP assistance, but that has since changed. Now, any employment earnings, including self-employed earnings, are based on a percentage basis. So after a certain level of income is reached, it is then determined how much will be deducted from each ODSP check, depending on how much is earned per month. I also was told that it is easier to be reinstated on ODSP if a job has come to an end.

This was one of the biggest problems for me many years ago when I went through a rough spot without employment. One of the biggest problems faced by people with disabilities is that we are unable to take just any type of job in order to get us through financially. We have to consider many factors that the average person doesn't even have to think about, and these factors change depending on each individual type of disability. Changes to the ODSP need to start with the amount of financial assistance. Too many people are falling through the cracks and are unable to make ends meet. In Thunder Bay, the low-income cutoff for a single person is $17,895, and for a family of four, it almost doubles to $33,711. A 2005 study indicated that about 14 percent of people in the city fall below the standard, which is barely enough to survive. The average single person with a disability who is on ODSP receives about $930 per month if living on his or her own. This figure is based on my own past experience. That's barely enough for people to pay rent to live in a respectable area. They can't buy food or pay their energy bills, which results in their relying on food banks and applying to programs designed to help those living on low incomes offset the cost of energy.

People with a disability who are solely dependent on ODSP and unable to work at a job with adequate pay need subsidized housing (i.e., rent geared to income) in order to live on their own, but the wait times are commonly nine months to a year before a subsidized unit becomes available. How can people in this situation make their circumstances better? This would be nearly impossible for most, unless they are able to further their education and get a financially secure career. What happens to those individuals who are unable to work at all because of their disability? There is no quality to life under those circumstances, so there is no incentive for them to try to find work and become independent. Independence and dignity are what everyone, disabled or not, wants. For people with a disability who cannot continue their education or who cannot work at all, the dream of having a better life becomes even more remote.

The entire ODSP needs to be revamped. For example, people who are receiving ODSP are eligible to receive eyeglasses, basic dental and drug coverage, and hearing aids. Special diet allowances, guide dog benefits, diabetic supplies, surgical supplies, and medical transportation may also be provided, depending on needs. The problem is that either these needs are not fully covered or there are too many rules and regulations, which render them useless in many situations. How can people on a fixed income scrape together enough money to pay a portion of the balance toward the necessary items they need that are not fully covered under the program when they are already unable to make ends meet?

Here's what eyeglass coverage typically includes: ODSP contributes $42 toward the cost of frames, and it covers the basic lenses, with absolutely no add-ons. I can't recall the last time I saw frames for $42. Even children's frames cost at least $60. As for the lenses, is it really a luxury to have glare-resistant or scratch-resistant coating added?

Drug coverage: In my experience, this has been one of the better coverage's. Rarely has something that my doctor has prescribed not been covered. In most cases, doctors will try to prescribe medications that are covered. Usually, many drug options are covered.

The dental plan: ODSP covers basic dental services, including fillings, X-rays, annual cleanings, and so on. However, I have a real problem with this plan. What happens when a person has some problems and needs more than basic dental services? For example, OI affects my teeth, which continually break for no apparent reason, just like my bones, so sometimes a tooth fracture requires more than just a filling. The tooth may need a crown and a post, at a cost of $1,000 or more. When I need dental treatment that isn't covered by ODSP, I've been told that I should go to Social Assistance and ask that agency to cover the cost. The plan did cover the cost for me once, but after that, I was told that they just do not have enough money in the budget to help me out again. ODSP then insists that the only option is to pull the tooth. This is archaic thinking at best, but for people under the ODSP dental plan, there really is little choice.

The last benefit that I have had experience with is hearing aids. Because I lost all of my hearing in my right ear and have some hearing loss in my left ear, I had no choice but to get a hearing aid. I was very pleased that ODSP paid for me to get a very small, state-of-the-art digital hearing aid that fit right into the ear canal, at a cost of $1,600.

As for the special diet allowance, guide dog benefits, diabetic supplies, surgical supplies, and medical transportation, I cannot comment on those services because I have not had a need for them.

I strongly believe that it's long overdue that we look at government programs such as this and revamp them to meet the realities of the twenty-first century.

Because I've always wanted to reach out and change things in my life, I have had a lot of experience with programs offered to people with disabilities to improve their situation, as well as to help them secure work, such as the Opportunities Fund through the Human Resources Development Centre (HRDC) and the Self-Employment Program through ODSP. One of the problems with these government programs is the number of rules and regulations, which can defeat the whole purpose of providing assistance. I went through these programs when I started both of my businesses. I received a great deal of assistance through ODSP's Employment Support Program. The help was tremendous, but I would like to shed some light on not only the positive but also the negative issues that I had experience with in hopes of making things better for those who apply in the future.

Please keep in mind that programs that I mention here may have been replaced with newer ones or perhaps been discontinued by the time you read this, so if you're in need of assistance, be sure to do your own research. Each person's circumstances are different, and this describes my own experiences with the system in Canada. I hope that by talking about my experiences, both the positive and negative, I can help other people who may be in a similar situation. I know how difficult life can be at times, and the unnecessary complications and often degrading processes can be depressing and embarrassing. I started to speak up at a very young age because I had to learn quickly how to be heard and how to be taken seriously. The spoken word has the power to hurt and the power to heal. When we learn to use it to our advantage, we can rise above our disadvantages and achieve greatness.

One of the greatest programs that the government in Ontario ever initiated is the Centre for Independent Living (CIL). This program was developed by consumers and the provincial government as a pilot project in 1994 to test a directly funded, self-managed model for adults with physical disabilities who need attendant services. For two years, the pilot was independently evaluated. This consumer-driven service model was so successful that in July 1998, the provincial government made it a permanent program and announced that it would be expanded to include seven hundred participants. New participants would be selected each year to receive funds in lieu of agency-delivered attendant services for which they would otherwise be eligible.

Self-Managed Attendant Services—Direct Funding is an innovative program that enables eligible adults with physical disabilities across Ontario to receive funds individually to recruit, manage, and pay for their own attendants. In essence, they become employers with all the associated responsibilities. The program is funded by the Ontario Ministry of Health and is administered by the CIL in Toronto in partnership with the Ontario Network of Independent Living Resource Centre.

This program is different from, and is intended as an option to, agency-delivered attendant service programs. In Ontario's delivered service models (supportive housing and attendant outreach services), an agency is the employer who provides attendant services to the consumer by sending attendants to the consumer's apartment or house. In the self-managed model, however, the consumers are the employers and take full responsibility for securing and managing their own attendants. There is no one else in charge. Adults with physical disabilities want to live independently and take charge of all aspects of their lives. They prefer to take full responsibility for the attendant services they need by employing their own attendant workers and managing their own funding. The option of self-management is supported by the Independent Living Movement, which promotes the independence that allows individuals to take responsibility for their lives, make choices, take risks, and participate fully in community life.

Anyone who is disabled, whether from birth or as the result of an illness or disease, can apply to this program. Based on extensive committee interviews, it is decided whether the applicant should be accepted. Once accepted, disabled individuals are allowed to hire someone for a certain number of hours per day to assist them with their activities of daily living (ADL). Attendant services provide consumer-directed physical assistance with routine ADL that the individuals would do for themselves if not for physical limitations. The consumers take responsibility for the personal decisions and training involved in their own assistance, which is provided by another person and involves positive human interaction.

When the number of hours a day and days per week the individual is allowed have been determined, a budget is set up to cover all of these costs. The services funded for any one individual will not exceed 180 hours per month (or 186 hours for months with thirty-one days) of attendant services (an average of six hours per day). The individuals have total control of whom they hire and exactly what they need assistance with for proper quality of life while living independently. The only stipulation is that they are not allowed to hire any family members, including husbands or wives. This is for the protection of the individuals, allowing them quality care without having to rely on family members or be taken advantage of by family members who may not have their best interests in mind.

All individuals accepted into the program must set up separate bank accounts under their name so that the funds can be deposited automatically each month. The individuals who are receiving the services must assume all responsibilities associated with being employers. These responsibilities may not be assumed by any other persons on behalf of the consumers. Management by another family member, or via power of attorney, is not permitted.

Attendant services do not include physiotherapy, rehabilitation, life-skills lessons, active nursing, socializing, and so on. Some of these professional services are provided through Community Care Access Centers. The Ministry of Health guidelines regarding monthly service maximums are currently under review, especially with respect to service levels for persons who require assistance in the maintenance of an airway or who use a ventilator at all times. When new policies come up, applicants and participants are advised about them. Except for cases defined in the ministry's guidelines, additional services or funding will not be granted.

Direct-funded services that provide individuals with the funds necessary to purchase their own attendant care services are an increasingly popular option in many jurisdictions. Alberta, Manitoba, Ontario, and Quebec have direct-funding projects. Attendant care services in the United States are also provided to people through Medicaid on a direct-funding basis.

The institutional approach was based on the assumption that people with disabilities are, for the most part, permanently incapacitated and are subsequently deemed incompetent. Increasing attention is being paid to the direct-funding approach, which focuses on the care and protection of people with disabilities, primarily in institutional settings. Over the last twenty years in particular, community living has replaced the institutional setting as the model of choice for delivering services to support people with disabilities. Early evaluations have shown that people with disabilities can live in the community.

Independent living has been defined by the Canadian Association of Independent Living Centers as "a process whereby disabled citizens achieve their desired individual lifestyles by assuming responsibility for the development and management of personal and community resources." Key principles of an independent living philosophy include autonomy and control by individuals over their own services. This differs from the traditional model, in which these decisions tend to be made by professionals. Independent living has been valued for its own inherent recognition of the autonomy and independence of people with disabilities.

# Chapter 20

## *Personal Reflections*

Regardless of the chaos around us and the challenges facing us, all that matters is what's in our hearts and souls. When life forces us to get rid of the clutter and the "busyness" that we so easily get caught up in, we begin to really live life as it is meant to be experienced. I believe that we come to earth having chosen the path that we will live, and that once we understand our personal journey, we can embrace life passionately. We are not on this earth necessarily to become a mother or a father, a husband or a wife. We are all here for the sole purpose of growing and learning and coming to know ourselves better.

Often, we become convinced that we must be married and have children to live life the "right way," or we think that we must achieve a certain level of education or a particular kind of job to feel successful and be respected. Deep down, we all know that these accomplishments don't actually matter as much as we think they do. What we really have to do in this life is **be accountable to ourselves.** How can we attain this? Looking deeply into the soul to find out what really makes us happy can give us a sense of why we are on this planet. What we often find is that we are unhappy doing the things that we think we believe, or have been told, that we ought to be doing. Each of us has something to offer, and we are all part of the big picture called life. Some of us need to learn and grow and achieve;

some of us don't feel the need in the same way. Not everyone is ready or able to grow at the same time or pace.

I have a strong belief in life after death. I believe that our time on earth is our chance to learn the many lessons that help our souls evolve so that we are able to leave our physical bodies one day and continue our journey elsewhere. I've also come to realize that living life with a disability never gets easier. There are always new obstacles and greater challenges. Living with a disability is the path that my life was meant to follow. The gift that I receive from my life is how I choose to deal with that challenge. One of my greatest motivators is the attitude that other people have toward me. When others think that they know what I can or cannot do, I rise above their expectations and strive to achieve the goals that are important to *me*.

Writing this book has been one of those goals.

I've been told that I'm an inspiration, but I've never thought that way. I'm just living my life and fulfilling the goals that are important to me. Living our earthly journey can be a challenge for all of us, but I've reached a point where I'm able to face the challenges and setbacks with the knowledge that I will get through them and be a better person for experiencing them. These are the building blocks. We all have a choice when faced with challenges. We can allow them to destroy our spirit, or we can use them to build character and inner strength. I read a quote once that touched my heart in a special way: "When you were born, you were crying and everyone around you was laughing. When you die, make sure you're the one that's laughing and everyone around you is crying."

What aggravates me more than anything is society's attitude toward people who are disabled or in some way different. This is one of the reasons for my wanting to write this book. I want people to become more knowledgeable and teach their children about diversity. I'm appalled by the rudeness of some adults, usually women, especially when they have children with them. These youngsters typically range from five years of age and up, and when such adults see me in a department store, a cashier's checkout, or even in a bank line, they look at me in sheer horror, immediately grab their children, and rush off. They act as if they've never seen anyone use a wheelchair before. This offensive and boorish behavior is totally unwarranted.

What does this behavior teach children? That people with disabilities should not be full participants in society? That people with disabilities should be kept indoors ... in locked rooms, with the curtains drawn? That people with disabilities don't have feelings, desires, or ambitions? For the life of me, I don't understand why some able-bodied adults are so uncomfortable in the presence of people with disabilities. Hasn't society yet evolved to the point of being inclusive and welcoming to all?

This negative and stifling attitude is precisely why it is difficult for people with disabilities to find and pursue careers and take on the normal responsibilities of functioning adults in society—almost as if people with disabilities are not supposed to grow up, have careers, live independently, participate in social activities, fall in love, get married, and have families of their own. The best way to end this attitude is to acknowledge it, talk about it with children, and be unafraid to help them at a young age realize that there are many people in this world who are different from each other. Being different doesn't make people with physical or cognitive challenges any less human. A disability is just "a state of mind." Just because I use a wheelchair to help me lead my life to the fullest doesn't make my heart and soul any different from yours.

Children are accepting and forgiving by nature; they just need to have their questions answered in the proper way and at the proper time. They should be taught to ask questions privately at home, not by yelling out in a crowd and laughing at things they may not understand. We can't let the ignorance and fear of adults be instilled in our children. I remember hearing someone once say that if a child has questions, the child should approach the person with the disability and not be afraid to ask about it. I think that whoever came up with that solution was completely unaware of what they were actually saying. It is not my job to teach everyone's child about diversity and good manners. I'm trying to live my life like everyone else, and I'm not here to explain to everyone, nor do I even feel that I have an obligation to explain why I may be different. It is a parental duty to help children accept differences; understand why those differences exist; and have the manners to interact with all humans, no matter how different they may be from themselves. Some days it's tough enough for me to get past the physical barriers, never mind having to teach strangers about OI, too.

I'm deeply moved when a child comes up and just starts talking to me, not about why I'm in a wheelchair, or why I'm small, or why my feet are so small, but just because he or she wants to talk. I know that such children have been taught the proper way to react and interact in society, and it gives me hope that we will one day accept each other unconditionally. If we speak to children at a very young age about the importance of accepting people with differences, we can avoid instilling unwarranted fears and ignorance in them.

No matter what other people have said or done, I've always known that I'm perfect the way I am. We are all perfect the way we are, which is the way God intended for us to be, and when children's souls are nourished properly, it doesn't matter what life might throw at them. I was probably nine or ten years old before I realized that I was physically different. What I mean is that I knew that I was different from other people, but I didn't know why it should matter. I used to ask my mother why people would stare at me. She always told me that they couldn't understand why someone who looked so healthy and beautiful was using a wheelchair. Her words never made me feel different from other people; in fact, they helped me become the strong and confident woman that I am today. What we believe as children determines who we become as adults. Being different in any way from what society tells us we should be opens the door to ignorance.

I have a great little test that may help each of us look at things with a different perspective and a fresh attitude. The next time you finish talking on the telephone with someone you've never met, think about how you treated that person. You probably judged that person by how the conversation went, not by looks, skin color, age, or maybe even disability. The next time you meet someone who may be different from yourself, remember to judge that person with closed eyes and an open heart. What you may find is that we really are not all that different from one another. There are many beautiful souls out there, and they come in all sorts of packages. You just need to take the wrapper off to find the gift that God has placed inside.

People often make assumptions about what they think someone with a disability is capable of doing. They somehow think that having a disability means not participating in anything that requires physical activity, even life, for that matter. My whole life I have struggled to overcome such ignorance. On one hand, I really don't care what others think I can, or can't, do, but on the other hand, I sometimes get so tired of the ignorance. Despite having OI, I've always participated in many physical activities: horseback riding, downhill skiing, snowmobiling, motorcycling, tobogganing, sledge hockey, swimming, and using the track at the gym to stay in shape. I love the outdoors, and camping, fishing, and boating have always been high on my list of activities because we did them quite often when I was a child. My disability has never prevented me from trying my hand at whatever interests me; in fact, that's probably what's driven me to even more accomplishments.

I have to be careful, but everything can be adapted if the will to participate is there. Sometimes, I have pushed the envelope and have ended up with a fracture or two, but that's been fine with me. I know what I feel comfortable doing, and I don't take risks. When I was growing up, Mom used to let me do whatever I wanted, within reason, but she later told me that she gave me her permission with her fingers crossed and a lump in her throat. I'm glad that my parents never held me back. They taught me to be aware of my condition and the consequences, but they also taught me to never let OI rule my life or dictate my choices.

So many people have preconceived notions of what my life must be like, but they are wrong. I have done more in my forty-five years than some people will do in a lifetime. I have always reached out and embraced life's precious opportunities. With all that I have had to deal with in my life, I know how precious life is. When I hear someone say, "Oh, I feel sorry for her," it makes me laugh because I'm the one feeling sorry for them for being so small-minded.

As I sit and watch Stan bowl with his Monday night league, I'm reminded about how content I am. I take the time to sit quietly and reflect upon my journey. Although there have been many bumps along the road, I would not change a single thing. The bumps made me appreciate the good times and realize how precious every moment is. I'm at a good place in my life, my heart, and my soul. I was blessed with the best parents that anyone could ever ask for; the most generous siblings; the most wonderful nieces and nephew; the most loving pets; the most genuine friendships and Stan, the only soul whom I have ever allowed to know the real me, with all of my faults, my weaknesses, my goals, my dreams, and my love.

I spent a long time wondering how I would end this book before I realized that there never really is an end. So if this book is the story of the first forty-five years of my life, what will I be able to write about the next forty-five years? To be continued ...

# Resources and Permissions

**Introduction**

A long time ago I met a very spiritual lady who recited the following quote to me. I never forgot those beautiful words, and I knew there and then that the quote was told to me for a reason. Never has the spoken word meant more to me than this quote does. I was unable to identify the author.

**Pg. 5** "Born a little more than perfect into a world a little less than perfect." (Author unknown)

The following quote came from the Internet, and I was unable to identify the author. When we think of our lives in reference to this quote, it helps us to understand life just a little bit more.

**Pg. 5** "May you have enough happiness to make you sweet, enough trials to make you strong, enough sorrow to keep you humble, and enough hope to make you happy." (Author unknown)

**Chapter 15: Personal Reflections**

**Pg. 64** I am honored to have been given permission by Mr. William N. Britton to include his poem "The Legend of Rainbow Bridge."

"The Legend of Rainbow Bridge": From the book, *The Legend of Rainbow Bridge* by William N. Britton. Published 1994. Copyright William N. Britton. Savannah Publishing c/o LikeMinds Press, Inc. 12203 Leona Lane Poway, CA 92064 www.legendofrainbowbridge.com Reprinted with permission of the author.

**Part Two: The Illness**
**Chapter 17: What is OI** and **Chapter 18: Treatment**

The Osteogenesis Imperfecta Foundation graciously granted permission to use their information in order to accurately convey technical and medical findings in both chapters 17 and 18 in Part Two.

Osteogenesis Imperfecta Foundation
804 W. Diamond Ave., Suite 210
Gaithersburg, MD 20878
Fax: 301-947-0456
Phone: 800-981-2663/301-947-0083
E-mail: bonelink@oif.org
Web: www.oif.org

**Chapter 19: My Goals and the System**

Information from the Centre for Independent Living was used to back up the views stated in this chapter on what I feel is one of the greatest programs that the government in Ontario ever initiated. The Centre for Independent Living (CIL) program was developed by consumers and the provincial government as a pilot project in 1994 to test direct funding as a self-managed model for adults with physical disabilities who need attendant services.

Centre for Independent Living in Toronto (CILT)
Direct Funding Program
205 Richmond Street West, Suite 605
Toronto, ON M5V 1V3
Phone: 416-599-2458/800-354-9950
TDD: 416-599-5077
Fax: 416-599-3555
Newsline: 416-599-4898
E-mail: dfinfo@cilt.cnd.com
Web: www.cailc.ca/cilt/index.htm

**Pg. 79** An article by Leith Dunick in *Thunder Bay Source*, October 12, 2007, discussed a 2005 study that indicated about 14 percent of people in the city fall below the standard income, which is barely enough to survive.

I read the following quote for the first time on the Internet. I was profoundly moved by the simplicity and beauty of how a meaningful life could be summed up. I was unable to identify the author of this beautiful statement.

**Pg. 83** "When you were born, you were crying, and everyone around you was laughing. When you die, make sure you're the one that's laughing and everyone around you is crying." (Author unknown)

# Reviews

"Heather Anderson has lived an extraordinary and courageous life, and I admire her resolve both as a human being and as a writer. In telling us her story, she provides a window into a world few of us could hope to know or understand ... and encourages our sensitivity, not just to the health issues and physical challenges of others, but to humanity in all its perseverance and breadth. Congratulations to her."

**Charles Wilkins, author of the national bestsellers**
***Walk to New York* and *The Circus at the Edge of the Earth***

"Heather Anderson tells a story of a life lived with fragile bones but a strong heart. Never willing to give up or to simply yield to the challenges placed in her path. Anderson's book relays the events of an inspiring life while bringing to the forefront crucial questions about health care in the twenty-first century. Even though Anderson encountered countless instances of discrimination, she was bolstered by a family that never held her back, and she refused to let herself be defined by her condition. Instead of pity or despair, her story carries a message of love and resiliency. Anderson is an inspiration to people of all heights!"

**Matt Roloff, author of *Against Tall Odds: Being a David in a Goliath World*, actor, farmer, inventor, and businessman, best known for starring with his family in the reality television program, *Little People, Big World***